The Time Of Your Life

THE

THE ULTIMATE

TIME OF

WOMEN'S GUIDE TO

YOUR

LIVING MIDLIFE BRILLIANTLY

LIFE

KAREN DAVIS

RETHINK PRESS

First published in Great Britain in 2019 by Rethink Press
(www.rethinkpress.com)

Cover image © Shutterstock: Steven Bourelle/MarySan/
Andrey_Popov

Contents

Introduction

'I started to become a woman at forty.'
—Robin Wright, fifty-two, actress

Welcome to the time of your life.

It's a phrase I'm sure we're all familiar with and it can be taken in so many ways. We might be having 'the time of our life' or it's just 'that time of life', but the challenge is as women, once we hit forty (and for some even earlier), we're on a path to a completely different kind of life. No question, no return tickets, we're in for a brand new ride that we probably didn't even see coming.

The problem is, we don't necessarily want it.

Many of us from forty onwards, whether we be fifty, sixty, seventy or older, still feel as though we are in our thirties. We're just a bit savvier. We quite liked our old lives, the one where the kids (if we had any) needed us, our figure could be kept under control with a couple of days' discipline, we could have a few bevvies and recover reasonably quickly and nothing really ached. All our friends were well, we were bowling along and life was pretty good. The challenge for women is that after forty, there's a whole load of other stuff that we need to know that we didn't know we would need to know when we were on Mumsnet or looking at skimpy bikinis to wear in exotic locations.

Welcome to this new life, and here's the thing: in midlife, you are going to have your greatest decade yet. I don't know the exact age this will start for you, but I've written this book so that you will find it. You will have the greatest decade of your life in midlife.

Forty is such a landmark in our culture and I've no idea why. We're female humans, we age, it is exactly what our life has marked out for us since birth. So what can we do?

Life up until now has been different for all of us, but there's no question that by the time we hit forty, we've started to understand some of its harshness. 'Stuff' has happened, be it divorce, money worries, death, hoo-ha with family, and it's all kicking off when our oestrogen is saying, 'Ta-ta'.

Did you think you had it tough as a stay-at-home mum or forging your career? Welcome to the evolved version of that.

The hard truth is that life after the age of forty shows us a much stronger scale of light and dark, and I'll run through why. Kids leave home, kids aren't doing well (this is so hard for mothers), parents and – how it hurts – friends pass on, money comes, money goes, partners come, partners go, we downsize and leave our family home where we had touchable memories of years together, we may need to find a new job, and somewhere in there is the menopause. It's not a great hand to be dealt.

Midlife is different for all of us, too. There is no one size fits all. One woman's easy menopause will be balanced by her friend's daily sweats and humiliation when she is wringing with damp in a meeting, remembering that she used to be the chick in the office who commanded corporate presentations with poise and verve. A happy partnership will be balanced by another woman's partner 'imaginatively' running off with their twenty-something colleague. A financially secure world will be balanced by someone else's hand-to-mouth existence.

But…

Midlife is an age when those of us with children will have more time because our children have left the nest. We'll all have a stronger sense of who we are because of the 'stuff' we've been through. But most importantly, we have a window in midlife to achieve dreams and ambitions that we couldn't get to when we were having a family or building a career. There is a potential ten-year 'Power Decade' that we can access to achieve everything we want to.

You'll need to be focused, you'll need some discipline, but midlife is the moment to put your life back on track, revisit what you wanted to achieve when you were in your twenties, decide if it is still important and put a plan into action to get the results. It really is now or never. Old age is in plain sight, so get the life you want now.

If you feel that some of your dreams have passed you by, that life hasn't quite turned out how you wanted it to, then this book will help you put it back on track while you still have the energy to do so and can handle the highs and lows of life. Yup, you'll get both, because midlife is a time when the truths of life are unveiled to you every day. You have to experience them because then you will really know who you are, when you are happy, you will find out what you want from life, and you will still have the time and energy to go and get it. You have a shining window of opportunity and you don't pass this way again.

As Robin Wright said, 'I started to become a woman at forty.' Welcome to womanhood – now let's go find your Power Decade.

1
Finding Your Power Decade

'Listen, the best advice on ageing is this: What's the alternative? The alternative, of course, is death.'
—Whoopi Goldberg, sixty-three, actress

Well, here we are, over forty and still alive. I'm not saying that lightly, I genuinely mean it. The sad truth is that not everyone makes it this far, so here's what we're going to do.

On hitting midlife, we are welcome to mourn the passing of our earlier years. Celebrate, remember all the fantastic, crazy things we did with our gorgeous, young, stretchy body. Hug our friends and family close – even have a small pity party, but after that, we'll put it away and not insult the memories of those who haven't made it this far by fearing what's to come. They would give anything to be in our shoes.

Many women (and one or two men) have contributed to this book, wanting to help you with the benefit of their knowledge, so you will be fine. First, we need to find your decade and recognise it when we see it, so let's make a start.

Why a decade?

Why not? It's a decent amount of time to change the course of our life.

Sometime between the age of forty and sixty-five you're going to know that the time has come to start your 'Power Decade'. Mine started at the age of fifty-two, but let's be flexible and see how far you can go.

In midlife, we're likely to see something happen to our immediate circle of friends. There will be those who stay in their era and seem unable to embrace the new things that come into the world. They are stuck. The DJs from their youth have moved from cutting-edge radio stations to easy-listening channels and they have followed them there. They're not listening to anything new, they're listening to exactly the same music as they were in their twenties, but they're now in their forties. This example works for so many other things, such as technology, newspapers, TV programmes – you name it, those who are stuck in a time warp don't embrace the new. They keep to the familiar in everything, and before long they'll be saying how dreadful young people are today.

You need to recognise if this is you, and if it is, you need to change. Now. You cannot find your Power Decade without embracing the new. People who are fixed in their ways are already preparing to retire in midlife. This book is all about preparing women to live amazingly and achieve more than ever in midlife.

We are going to get tech savvy (if we aren't already), we are going to mix with all ages of people, we are going to actively make incredible friendship circles with people we don't even know yet. We are going to try new things, we are going share our skills, we are going to be kind and help people, some of whom we may never see again. Wow. And this is only Chapter One.

We need a decent amount of time to achieve the life we really want because it is likely to involve some fundamental changes. We'll need to put blocks in place first and grow into it; we can't become as awesome as Michelle Obama overnight. Even Mrs Obama took time to become as awesome as she is now, so we're giving ourselves the years to make it happen. Ten years, and then we'll see where we go from there. Sound reasonable?

Understand that we are not talking about a midlife crisis. A midlife crisis comes about when we realise our youth is over and old age and even death are now touchable. That's a horrible sentence to write. Who wouldn't have a midlife crisis thinking that? Midlife crisis is about trying to regain what is gone, to capture some of the aspects of being young again, and it is a non-forward-thinking process; it is a process of denial. If you decide you want a sports car, you crack on, but when your knees won't get you out of it terribly fast and you're looking less than elegant as you hoist yourself from the seat, don't say I didn't warn you.

Our Power Decade is light years away from a midlife crisis. It's got nothing to do with the word 'crisis', it's all to do with the word 'power'. We are re-imagining, nay, embracing our midlife years as a place where we feel brilliant, thrilled not to be dealing with the challenges of our twenties and thirties, in complete (well, almost) control of the challenges that midlife throws our way while proactively achieving all that we wanted to do. That's quite a different story.

Recognising your power decade

This is the fun bit, and I genuinely mean that as there are a few different forces at play. There are three ways to recognise when your Power Decade is about to start:

- When you are physically ready
- When you are mentally ready
- When you feel great about your midlife self

There, that was simple.

Your life is completely unique. Your set of physical, mental and material circumstances as you arrive at the age of forty are different to anyone else's and that's why only you, no one else, can recognise when the moment is right to launch your Power Decade.

Physical health

We're going to spend a reasonable amount of time on this because it is absolutely key. You cannot have a

Power Decade unless you are doing everything you possibly can to be fit and healthy. That doesn't mean that you aren't battling some serious physical challenges, you may well be. What it means is that you are at the peak of physical health *for you*.

Your Power Decade is going to be demanding. You want it that way because you are seeking to have achievements as the outcome. The truth is that none of us are getting any younger, so we need to do everything we can to ensure that we have the energy, stamina and health to do what we want to do. Remember, your Power Decade is a choice: you have chosen to do this. As such, you have agreed to get yourself in top shape. Why wouldn't you?

There are two types of health challenges. The first relates to lifestyle choices we've made – diet, exercise, ciggies, booze, etc – and the second relates to those that happen to us whether we like it or not, like the menopause. We'll discuss both of these types of challenges, but start by making decent choices on the bits you can control and recognising how much you are being held up by health issues outside of your control. If you're having a challenging menopause, I can guess exactly where you'd like to tell me to stick my Power Decade until you are through it and out the other side. If your menopause is relatively easy, you may feel that you can start earlier. Who knows when your menopause will start and end? By forty you may be through it, or, like me, you may be fifty-six and there are signs it's still not finished with you yet.

Be realistic. You're a grown up now, so be honest about the bits of your physical health you can change and those you can't. We'll look at this in a lot more depth in Chapters Two and Three.

Mental health

To undertake a Power Decade, we need to be up for it. We need to have come to the realisation that life hasn't quite turned out how we wanted it to, that if we left this mortal coil now, our legacy as it stands today wouldn't be what we wanted it to be.

This can be a depressing thought process, but we all need to go through it. I did, even though I spent time justifying to myself why I hadn't achieved what I wanted to. I'm not sure why I took quite so long pondering it as the solution remains the same: to change, to make the things I wanted to happen, happen.

This is the reason we need the Power Decade. Even though I knew some things needed changing, I wasn't able to do it for many years until I had this window of time. For me, I still had to get my kids to college, and until that process had started, my mental energies were on them, not on me. My career hadn't gone as meteorically as it could have because I wanted to take my kids to school and put them to bed at night, so I made a trade-off. A happy trade-off, but it did mean I didn't achieve career-wise what I thought I could. Of course, I could have been completely wrong, but I wanted to try; I wanted to see just how far I could have gone.

For you, it could be that you are going through a divorce which is taking all your energy. You could be looking after ageing relatives, stuck in a dead-end job, struggling financially – all manner of things could be going on in your life that need to be put to bed before you can focus on you.

And this is another challenge. The reason we need our Power Decade is likely to be because we have put others before ourselves for quite some time while our needs and desires took a back seat. A Power Decade is about righting this; it is now all about us and that's quite a switch to make in our heads, from being second (or lower) in the pecking order when it comes to allocating our time to being top. We need to deal with this as well, so we'll talk about it in detail in Chapter Four.

How you feel about yourself

In short, this bit is all about confidence. We cannot have a Power Decade of achievements if we don't feel great about ourselves. Physical health and mental health are strong forces, but we also need to feel fabulous.

This may have eluded you in recent years. I went through a time of wearing just four boring outfits as I couldn't fit into anything else, and with a wardrobe full of clothes, I couldn't bring myself to buy any new ones. I didn't feel fabulous during this time, but I felt fabulous when I lost weight and could wear my lovely clothes again.

Feeling great about ourselves is tied up with complex issues. It's about how we look, how we feel, how we think others perceive us, and so many other thoughts we have about ourselves, but I'm simply going to talk you through a makeover of skincare, makeup and hair (see Chapter Four). It could be that the last time you really examined how you present yourself to the world was in your twenties or thirties, and your face is now a whole lot different to then.

So, there you have it: physical health, mental space and confidence. Let's get these three under our belt to set ourselves up in the best possible way to get the most out of our Power Decade.

2
Health Issues We Can Control

'Old age ain't no place for sissies.'
—Bette Davis, 1908–1989,
legendary Hollywood actress

Let's focus on what's really important to get the most out of midlife, and number one is our health.

Before we turned forty, being healthy was pretty easy. We chose to put on weight, we chose to keep slim. We chose to join a gym or not, embrace yoga or not, go to our smear tests or not. The odds were with us and our young bodies.

That currency is now on a ticking clock and we have to look at our health a bit more seriously, because good health in midlife is essential. It sets us up for the future and, trust me, more health issues seem to come up as we get older. Every decade will bring new challenges, so if we haven't looked after our health properly before, now is the moment to re-evaluate and decide our plan of action.

Don't think it'll never happen to you – this train is coming. It's a bit like buying Apple shares in the eighties. No one knew what they'd be worth now, but I certainly wish I'd invested. Health is the same. We have no idea what an investment in our health will be worth to us in later life, but you're going to have to trust me on this one. Do it. No need to thank me.

Before forty:

- We haven't been invited to have mammograms
- We exercise and see reasonably quick results
- Our sex drive peaks, usually in our twenties

Now that's all about to change and it can be a shock. Our bodies have pretty much done what we've told them to since we were teenagers, but now? Now it's time to take a tight rein on matters.

Basically, after forty we need to have a care as nothing will bounce back like it did before. We can think of it like a salary. Every month from now on, we're going to make health decisions based on our diet, exercise and how we take care of ourselves. If we put effort into the 'Bank of Me', we should be OK; if we make no effort at all, we're likely to be in overdraft. In other words, if we stay fit and eat well, our health should be good; if we don't, there may well be some obstacles to overcome. No one says that anything is a given. We may live incredibly well and still get something nasty, but there's no question that if we've taken care of ourselves, we'll be in a better place to fight it. Do nothing and we're in a more difficult place to mount the counteroffensive.

So let's look at the aspects of our health that we can control.

Nutrition

There are three aspects to our diet from the age of forty:

• What we should eat for our health

• What we should not eat for our health

• The amount we can eat

One of the things that really fascinates me is the change in what we should eat for optimum health as a midlife woman. Turns out that salmon and hummus are to be our new best friends – who knew? Pop in a few eggs, a truck load of veg, some olive oil and we're pretty much there. OK, there's a bit more to it than that, but here's the thinking.

Dr Marilyn Glenville is the former president of the Food and Health Forum at the Royal Society of Medicine, a registered nutritionist, psychologist, author and popular broadcaster who obtained her doctorate from Cambridge University. To me, she is an international expert on women's health through nutrition and has had some incredible results. Phytoestrogens, omega 3 fatty acids, vitamins B, C, D and E, magnesium and calcium are her backbones of the midlife woman's diet, and here's why.

Phytoestrogens

These seem to be key for helping alleviate the symptoms of menopause. In the Far East, women have minimal and often no menopausal symptoms, whereas in the West it's a real issue. Likewise, breast cancer is not the major killer in the East that it is in the West – why?

Scientists have concluded that this is to do with the plant hormones called phytoestrogens. Don't ask me why, but they have. Phytoestrogens occur naturally in soya – why is it always something like soya? Why is it not occurring naturally in lemon shortbread? They also lower cholesterol as well as offering low-level disease prevention. So, you need to start including fermented soya, sage, flaxseeds and alfalfa in your diet. Crack on.

Omega 3 fatty acids

My mother used to chug down the evening primrose oil in an effort to get more omegas, but it's not quite as straightforward as that. You need to give yourself a test to check on your omega levels. You can do it at home, but blood will be involved. I've included test kit details at the back of the book.

Omega 3 fatty acids lubricate the body and help with dry skin, hair, nails, tiredness and a whole host of things that we don't want in our lives. They also have an anti-inflammatory action on the body so we really need these, but in the right quantities. Omegas can come from a whole host of foods – salmon, mackerel, sardines, caviar if you've got a decent budget and a taste for the stuff, as well as plants such as flaxseed. Test your levels and add these into your diet two to three times each week. Go on, it's good for you and calming for the menopause.

Vitamins B, C, D and E

These four vitamins are great for midlife women.

Vitamin C helps our immune system, prevents illness and encourages good health in general, including helping to prevent stress incontinence (a potential side effect of the menopause which none of us like).

Vitamin E is key because, although most women fear breast cancer, our actual biggest killer is heart disease. Vitamin E is meant to help resist heart attacks and it's supposedly more effective than aspirin.

B vitamins help manage stress which can be very real in menopause.

Vitamin D helps calcium be absorbed by the body which is essential to help keep osteoporosis at bay.

Magnesium and calcium

These help, in conjunction with other foods, to counter mood swings and build strong bones.

You can get all of the above from your diet or from quality supplements, depending upon your choices, but I recommend you make sure you're getting them. It will make all the difference to your health.

Your weight

'Many times you look in the mirror and you don't even recognize your own self because you got lost – buried – in the weight that you carry.'
—Oprah Winfrey, sixty-four, media phenomenon

Your weight. I'm really sorry, but you need to try to get into a healthy weight range. It is a cornerstone to living midlife well and cutting down your risk factors for heart disease and cancer, and it makes exercise easier so that you have more energy for your life. About 50% of us midlife women are obese – not just fat, obese – and we know that we got this way because life just took its toll on our discipline. I say this with love in my heart, not because I judge how you look; that's not of interest to me. It may be to you, but not to me. At this point you need to be a healthy weight. It needs to be done. There, I've said it, so you choose what you want to do. No hard feelings.

Let's talk about why eating well (whatever your weight) is crucial to a happy midlife. Your metabolism starts declining in your forties pretty much like this:

If you are inactive and want to maintain your weight:

- Twenty-five to thirty years old – eat 1,800 calories per day

- Thirty to fifty years old – eat 1,700 calories per day

- Fifty onwards – eat 1,600 calories per day

If you are active and want to maintain your weight:

- Twenty-five to thirty years old – eat 2,400 calories per day

- Thirty to fifty years old – eat 2,200 calories per day

- Fifty onwards – eat 2,000 calories per day

What does this tell us? If we exercise, we get to eat more food. Yummy. But if you want to lose weight, consider this. There are 3,500 calories in 1 lb of fat, so if you are inactive from the age of fifty onwards, you'll have to go down to 1,100 calories per day, which is not much, to be honest. You'll then lose 1–2 lbs per week. The excitement…

If you have to lose weight, do it as early as possible, ideally around the age of forty. Get into shape and get your weight under control. Be the correct weight for your height and build. This has nothing to do with fatism, nothing to do with looks, nothing to do with anything but your intrinsic health. I only care about your ratio of lean muscle tissue/bone to fat. End of.

Being overweight increases your risk of these illnesses and diseases:

- **Type 2 diabetes** – you can go blind or lose limbs from this. In the UK there are twenty amputations of lower limbs per day due to type 2 diabetes, an utterly preventable disease.

- **High blood pressure** – puts pressure on your heart, can cause kidney or heart disease.

- **Heart disease and strokes** – I'm sure you know these aren't good.

- **Cancer** – increased risk of breast, colon and endometrium cancers. None of these are nice.

- **Osteoarthritis** – one in three of us is getting osteoporosis, so why compound the problem?

- **Fatty liver disease** – could lead to liver failure.

- **Kidney disease** – yup, pretty sure we need kidneys in midlife, so best to keep them.

Our health is likely to get worse as we get older, fact, but even as a midlife woman, you may have limited knowledge of the real impact of the above, so you won't know how bad they can be. Just trust me, they're bad, so I recommend you avoid them by nutting up and losing the weight.

There are many ways to lose weight and I'm sure you're bright enough to understand the choices. I'll make a few suggestions of my own at the end of the book, but the best advice is to find a way that works for you and get on with it. Just get it out of the way.

Lecture over.

Alcohol

'The most important thing I learnt was that "the first drink does the damage". If I didn't have the first one I wouldn't want the next one.'
   —Anne Robinson, 2001 from *Memoirs Of An Unfit Mother*

It's wine o'clock! God, don't you love that phrase? Whether we're coming out of a stressful day at work, off the back of eighteen hours straight with kids or it's the start of the weekend, wine o'clock is for many of us a highlight of our day. Swathes of blogs, newspaper columns, cards and 'fun' gifts testify to the 'mummy wine' phenomenon. I've had 'whole bottle in a glass' gifts from my kids and I've embraced the fabulous culture around drinking with groups of female friends.

But...

That now has to slow down, a lot. And in my case, it stopped.

I completely get that after stress, wine is fantastic. The pressure valve lifts and those first few definitely give us confidence in a roomful of people. Years ago, I asked someone from a management centre why all the women I knew had a bevvy when they got back from work, whereas in my mother's era it was all cups of tea.

'It's to do with the time that you have available to release pressure,' he said. 'Years ago, life wasn't this fast. There were no mobiles, no internet, only three TV channels, and when you got home you had time for the ritual of tea to do its work in alleviating stress.

These days, no one has that time, so we're all after an instant, fast release of the pressure valve, and alcohol does that.'

I assume drugs do the same, but I look so straight that no one has ever offered me any so I wouldn't know.

I associate alcohol with fun, holidays, treats, some of the best nights of my life, but I know, deep in my heart, that alcohol isn't good for me, which is why I've stopped. I drink about a dozen times per year now, but is this sacrifice worth it?

In your sixties, your lifestyle choices start catching you up. And this is one of those lifestyle choices.

Alcohol is fundamentally a poison. Oh yes, one that's watered down and with a fair amount of sugar in it, but don't try to get away from the fact that it is a poison. It also isn't great for women. It affects us faster than men and is a real ingredient in increasing our chances of breast cancer. It contains a shed load of calories, so our weight will be affected and our type 2 diabetes risk goes up as well. Not only that, it has an impact on the way others view us, too.

I was pulled up short when my son gave me the whole bottle in a glass gift. He saw me as someone who was a serious drinker, but I'd been kidding myself that I was nowhere near that stage. I was wrong.

You see, the alcohol thing creeps up. It's one or two glasses at the weekend, then a bottle between two isn't enough so we've bought two bottles for the evening, and we might as well finish them. And then there's a third in the fridge, 'just in case'. We're now on a bottle a night and it's become like orange squash to us, and suddenly we're functioning alcoholics because we're at least thinking about that first glass earlier and earlier in the day. That moves on to a craving, but we're still getting up and all our work gets done, so we don't realise how bad the cycle is that we're in.

In 2018, the UK's professional medical journal, *The Lancet*, said there is 'no safe level of drinking alcohol'. Sure, I read the press stories that tell us a glass of red wine a day is great, but if it's that restorative, why don't doctors prescribe it? Why isn't it doled out on the cardiac ward at the local hospital? Because it's a poison, that's why. Alcohol is expensive, indisputably linked to a whole range of diseases for women, disrupts sleep, throws our body out of chemical balance and doesn't do much for our brain or skin. It sometimes makes us not very nice people, and definitely enables us in making bad choices at the time.

I suggest that you seriously reconsider your intake. I'm not a party pooper, but really, from forty onwards, alcohol should be for high days and holidays with no place in your weekday fridge. And a high day is not Saturday night or a meal out, either; it's a birthday, a friend's birthday, Christmas. Don't lie to yourself, you're a big girl now.

Smoking

This is also *very* bad. If you've ever smoked seriously, you'll know there are certain times that a cigarette seems like the most fantastic thing on earth, in the same way that a glass of wine has occasions when it completes the memory. But, of course, in exactly the same way that we can drink alcohol as a perfunctory habit, so can we consume cigarettes in day-to-day humdrumness. Both alcohol and ciggies are addictive, both cause terrible harm to the body, both can result in death, both are legally obtainable from any supermarket.

As with alcohol, if you're a smoker, I urge you to give up. Not only could cigarettes be lethal to your health, they (and alcohol) make menopause symptoms so much more pronounced.

Have you seen anyone with lung challenges in old age? It's not a pretty sight. I've seen someone die of pneumonia, and that wasn't a day to pop in the memory bank to cherish later. Smoking will also limit what you can do now. Exercise is more difficult, as is playing with any grandchildren you may have, and even people who are significant in your life can be turned off by the smell, but if you carry on smoking, you'll never know many opportunities you've missed. At my hairdresser's, there are two people who blow dry my hair pretty well, but I go with the non-smoker as I don't like the smell of cigarettes on the other stylist, so she's missed out on business, gossip and tips.

No one ever says, 'Oooh, you're a smoker, just what I wanted', unless they're running medical trials for a new drug. I suppose at least they might pay you to test for them, but that's the only benefit I can see. Your children might not leave your grandchildren with you because you smoke; you might not be asked to dinner because the host is dead against it; you could miss out on a potential partner because it's a deal breaker for them. For all of us non-smokers, these issues never even enter our heads, which puts us at an advantage.

Finally, have you seen the cost of cigarettes these days? OMG, I could not believe it! When I did smoke (and that wasn't much and not for long), they were

£1.72 for twenty. When I last looked, that same box cost £11–£12 – that is unbelievable. If you drink and smoke, you could be spending £50–£100 per week on stuff that's killing you; that's over £5k per person per year. If you're intent on killing yourself via smoking, I suspect Dignitas would be cheaper in the long run.

I don't need to say more. Make your own choice, but if you want an incredible, amazing, fulfilling Power Decade, choose to live well.

A helping hand

I'm not unfeeling, so I'm going to help you lower the amount you drink or smoke until you stop altogether, because if I can do it, anyone can. Here's how we're going to do it.

1. Download and print the Monthly Quit Chart from my website (at www.toyl.co.uk/pages/the-book, see also at the back of this book) and put it somewhere you'll see it as your first step. This is really going to help you. On the fridge, the bedside table, or anywhere you'll actually see it a couple of times a day, but *not* folded up in your handbag. You'll forget it.

2. Get in the mood to give up. If you're mentally not there, it's not going to happen. Google all the reasons alcohol or cigarettes are not helping you be fantastic and write them down on the chart. This is your why. Make your why really strong; a weak why isn't going to work.

3. Think about your reaction to giving up alcohol or cigarettes. Are you horror struck at the thought? If so, perhaps you're more dependent than you realised.

4. Pick a date (soon, not next year) and write it at the top of the page. Tick box number one if you make it through the day with no alcohol or cigarettes. What you're looking for is momentum, ie a block of three, four, five days without alcohol. Then you're likely not to want to break the run.

5. At some point, you're likely to say, 'Sod it'. At this moment, all your good intentions will fly out the window and the temptation will be right there in front of you. Here's my advice. If you can possibly reach into the depths of your memory, remember why you stopped. If you can, give it ten minutes before you give in. Call a friend for a catch up *now* as distraction is an amazing way to stop cravings. And cravings are just that. Honestly, hand on heart, if you can resist for ten minutes, they will likely be gone. The ten-minute rule is key to remember.

6. If you do give in, have a sip or a single drag and then stop. Put the cigarette out. Put the glass of wine down. Think. Give it a few minutes. What was it like? Had you built it up in your mind to be something that the reality didn't deliver? The glass or cigarette is still there, you've made your decision, but just wait. How do you feel? Do you still want it? Has the single sip or drag helped and stopped the thought that you 'can't have it'? If so, put some cling film over the top of the glass – I'm not saying you can't have it – and pop it back in the fridge. Leave the cigarette in the ashtray. After another five minutes, do you still want it? If not, leave it. It won't go off overnight. If you still want it, have it, but try to stop after one.

7. One type of alcohol is not better than another. A gin and slimline tonic is less calorific than a vat of wine, but it's alcohol and it's not good for you. You're not on a calorie thing here, you're on an alcohol thing.

8. Don't beat yourself up. This is a work in progress, and even I give in sometimes. What matters is that the balance has changed incredibly so that I now wouldn't class myself as a drinker at all. Moderation rather than being a killjoy is what you are after with the booze here (your life will be better without cigarettes altogether). Give it up, and then

be judicious about when you use alcohol in the future. It's for your health.

I set up a reward system for myself. If I managed not to drink for an entire month, I bought myself a full-body massage. If I failed, I couldn't have it. Think about what might work for you and do reward yourself. You can afford it now you're not buying Echo Falls or twenty Benson and Hedges every night.

There's another benefit as well. I got back hours in an evening when I was sparkly-eyed awake. Instead of a wine stupor coming on around 8.30–9pm, I could be productively awake until 10.30pm. Doing something with that time really helped and I tried to be as creative as possible with it. We'll talk about that more in Chapter Six.

Exercise

'I started going to the gym to get fit for a movie about climbing a mountain, which we filmed for two months solid, and now I'm addicted to it.'
—Sheila Hancock, eighty-five, actress

This is essential. Non-negotiable.

Exercise and fitness hold the formula to alleviating so many ailments as we get older. Proven many times over. Fact.

It's no coincidence that so many kids are obese now that school sport is almost at zero. Private schools have massive sports facilities and programmes – do you know why? They recognise the health benefits, both physical and mental, of exercise and have the funds to do something about it. State schools also recognise this but just don't have the freedom to necessarily address this, plus the government may have sold off their sports fields which doesn't seem such a good idea now.

Here are the reasons exercise is essential to your wellbeing as a midlife woman:

It prevents osteoporosis. I don't actually need to go much further than this, do I? The thinning of our bones as we get older is highly likely. This will make them weak. This means when we fall (and remember, 50% of us will fall after the age of fifty), we're more likely to break a hip. Break a hip when we are much older and we may well be on a cycle to getting pneumonia and not coming out of hospital at all. Broken hips are a well-known risk factor for premature death. You may think this is an exaggeration, but trust me.

Many older people are on this cycle – ask any of your friends who are carers.

Weight-bearing exercise massively helps keep bones strong, so do more of this good stuff.

It controls weight. From the age of around thirty-five, we start to lose muscle at the rate of 0.5% to 1% per year. This is bad. Muscle keeps our bones in alignment, helping us have the energy and the strength to do physical tasks throughout our day. Even better, muscle is the engine that burns fat.

If you weigh 10 stone and have a goodly proportion of muscle, you will be able to eat far more calories with no weight gain than someone who is 10 stone and has a much lower proportion of muscle. You really want muscle in your life.

It fights all other diseases. Almost every disease you can think of has less chance of flourishing if your body is fit.

It alleviates back pain. What a misery this can be, and yet so much back pain can be alleviated by exercise.

It helps us keep up. Do you want to be old before your time? Exercise enables us to keep up much better with kids and grandkids and enjoy the time we spend with them rather than being exhausted or telling them we'll catch them later.

It tones your arms. How quickly do you want to be covering up bingo wings?

It tones the tops of your legs – ditto, but replace bingo wings with cellulite.

It releases endorphins. We're not getting any from alcohol or cigarettes anymore, so let's get the free ones with exercise that make us feel great.

It makes us feel better. Not at the time. At the time, we may feel horrible, but after exercise, we feel great.

Few of us are natural gym bunnies who cannot wait to get into a plank position, but the benefits to our health of doing exercise are so enormous, we need to include it in our daily routine like brushing our teeth. It's just a thing we do. The fundamental key, the golden goose of exercise, the way forward for all of us midlife ladies, is weight-bearing exercise so we are going to start with this. Are we going to pile on muscle? I sincerely hope so. Are we going to look like a body builder? Absolutely not. It's almost physically impossible for you or me to achieve that look – we're not dedicated enough.

Why are we starting with weight-bearing exercise? Because of the osteoporosis threat and because people with muscle burn more fat than those who weigh the same but have less muscle. We want to be fat-burning machines to protect ourselves against future weight gain.

I know what it's like going into a gym full of fitties and working around the blokes to get at the weights. I know the looks they give us midlife women, thinking we haven't got a clue about what we are doing and wondering why we are in their workspace. But here's the thing. I'm actually an ex-fitness instructor (another life) and I'm telling you that virtually all the men on the free weights are doing their workouts wrong, so don't let them intimidate you.

I spoke to Geraldine Tuck, a woman I've known since she graduated from university who is massively committed to getting people moving. Geraldine is the ukactive strategic development director and is constantly working with partners to create new concepts to get us to exercise. She also lobbies the government to move exercise up the agenda and redid her personal trainer qualification in 2018, just so she could stay current.

I interviewed her about midlife women exercising and this is what she said.

'Women often lose their way with exercise. They get caught up in so much of daily life that this often drops off their agenda, but, in fact, research shows that 50% of women in midlife are obese. Not overweight, obese. That automatically increases their risk of breast cancer by 20%, so from one in eight to one in six. Not only that, there are thirteen common cancers where your risk is increased just by being overweight, and that's before we get on to bone density.'

Geraldine pointed out that women up to the age of fifty-four pretty much exercise like younger women, but after fifty-four we seem to get into group exercise much more, favouring Pilates, tai chi and yoga over impact-bearing classes, which are so important for bone strength.

'Ideally, I'd like midlife women to be doing a brisk walk every day. Not so they're sweating, but definitely one that elevates their heart rate. I'd also like them to do two sessions each week that helps build their bone strength such as running, hand-held weight classes, in the gym using weights, or even press ups using knees to start at home. Without your skeleton being strong, your health is in a really difficult place.'

We also talked about why women put exercise off.

'I think it's really hard for your younger self to understand the benefits of exercise fully. It's hard, in a world of instant gratification, to understand the benefits that an exercise programme that you start now can give you in twenty years' time. It genuinely is a magic pill for so many ailments and diseases, but it needs effort. So many of us put these choices off because they do require effort and time out of our day, but they are so worth it. We also forget how great we feel after exercise as those endorphins are released. Exercise helps with mental health, stress, relaxation, metabolism and has so many other benefits, while there are also so many ways to exercise that are really enjoyable. You just need to find one.'

And this is true. You may hate the idea of exercise, but you never feel worse for having done it. It makes you feel amazing. Virtuous. Smug. And it really helps your metabolism. I tell you now that a fifty-year-old with good muscle density and strength will burn way more calories by standing up than her twin with less muscle doing the same thing. Muscle burns more calories than fat just by being – fact.

What do we want? Muscle!

How do we want it? With strong bones!

I accept that this isn't much of a chant, but strong bones and muscle are our first ports of call for a healthy midlife.

Give it a go.

3
Health Issues We Can't Control

'Our health always seems much more valuable after
we lose it.'
  —Anon

The challenges we'll face

Let's start with a cheery list of the key challenges coming our way for the next few decades.

Forties

The **perimenopause** (the time shortly before the
menopause) is right up there as the number-one

bit of health fun in this decade and it's the biggest sign to most women that they are moving through life. It's completely different to anything we've experienced before; it's a rite of passage into a new part of our lives.

It's highly likely you will become perimenopausal in your forties, which can be the most challenging bit of the whole thing. There are libraries of books and blogs on this subject, so all I will say is that whatever anyone has told you it would be like, your menopause will be completely individual to you.

Your **metabolism** is likely to change. OK, when I say change, I don't mean that it's going to speed up so that you can eat more chocolate cake. It's likely to slow down by up to 5% per decade from now on, which makes weight gain a real possibility.

Being overweight is just not good for health. For women, if you're apple shaped (like me) and all your fat is around your stomach, the odds are you are more likely to be susceptible to heart issues. Lose the fat for your health, not for your wardrobe. Get into the normal range of body fat and stay there. It's key for your wellness going forward. Not easy, but it's something to put your head down and crack on with (see the section on nutrition in the previous chapter). It's now a non-negotiable. Sorry, I don't like giving you non-fun tasks, but I'm not going to lie to you.

Hair loss. This is a great list, isn't it? Hair can thin, even in your early forties. Don't panic, there are options that we'll discuss in Chapter Four, and its hair loss *everywhere*, if you get my drift.

Brain fog. I'm tempted to put the crying with laugher emoji here as this is so real. Don't beat yourself up about it if you increasingly go into rooms and can't remember what you went in for. It happens. I'm told that memory function improves after menopause, but it'll get worse before it gets better, if it does get better.

Bladder control, or lack of it. If you've had kids, then 'down there' has been under assault and you may well start sneezing and getting a surprise. Around this time, I stopped going on the trampoline with my kids as I didn't think Tena Lady pants were the look I wanted to rock in my forties. I'm happy to leave that to my eighties and then wear them with pride. You need to get into pelvic floor exercises fast. Do them daily. I've got an Elvie (see end of book for details) and it has helped but honestly, it's a device that you don't need if you're more motivated than me to do pelvic floor exercises. The key exercise is to squeeze your back passage tight and move that feeling forward to your pelvic floor. Start at the back, move the squeeze forward, from back passage to front passage, if you get my drift. Do it as often as you can, but at least 10-15 times each day, slowly.

Muscle loss. After the age of thirty-five, we start to lose muscle at the rate of 0.5% to 1% per year, so if you're reading this book at the age of forty, you're already into at least 2.5% muscle loss. You may not think this is key, but it is *crucial* to your midlife health as a woman. Resistance training should be put on your 'to do' list.

Muscle burns more calories than the same weight of fat, supports your bone structure, keeps you well. I can't talk to you enough about the benefits of muscle as a midlife woman, but I hope you'll be a convert by the end of the book. See your bum? How saggy do you want it to be? I know, that was a low blow, but really, I just wanted your attention. I actually want you to keep your muscles toned for the benefit of your health.

Fifties

Lucky you, it's time for your first **mammogram**! At the age of fifty, every woman in the UK is invited for a mammogram, and then they're invited every three years. Diarise it and go; think of those who regretted the fact that they didn't and give thanks that we are lucky enough in the UK to get this on the NHS. Other countries will differ in what's available, but do seek out a mammogram every three years from your fifties on. Go earlier if you think there might be an issue.

Will it hurt? I'm going to go with what the midwife said to me:

'There will be discomfort.'

It's easier if you have larger breasts, but it's nothing worse than a smear. Mine takes place in the back of a truck in the library car park – lovely.

Osteoporosis. Over the age of fifty, almost half of women will have a hip, wrist or vertebrae fracture during the rest of their lifetime. Frankly, I'm keen to avoid any of these. If you have history in your family of osteoporosis then man up and put 'strength training' on your to-do list. It is a drug-free way of improving your bone density.

Urinary tract infections. You may well get more urinary tract infections (UTIs) which are common after menopause. You're getting all the fun, aren't you?

Post menopause, or rather, just menopause, because you should be out the other side at some point in your fifties and (allegedly) the brain fog will lift and you'll feel a whole lot better.

Sixties

Bone density scan. The NHS doesn't offer free bone scans, but it is definitely worth having one. Loads of places do offer them, so I recommend you have one done every couple of years. You are looking for signs of osteoporosis because there is quite a lot you can do to help yourself if you have it, but you need to know early. I've suggested private bone scan suppliers at the end of the book.

Sensory decline. Your five senses (taste, touch, hearing, sight and smell) may well decline in your sixties. Just be sensible. Go to sight tests, get your hearing tested and keep yourself well.

Life choices catch up. Bit of a bugger this one, which is why I suggest that you start moving to a healthier lifestyle from forty onwards, or as young as possible if forty has already been and gone. It will pay you back massively.

If you want to use me as an example, my lifestyle choices started catching up with me at the age of fifty-five in a spectacular way, so I went full goodie-two-shoes immediately. I now hardly drink alcohol, I never smoke and my diet is exemplary. These days I settle down with a cup of tea and trawl online shoe, bag and clothing stores with an increased budget from the savings on vino (yes, I know, how much was I drinking?).

Cancer. The risk of endometrial, ovarian, colon, breast and lung cancers increases, with 50% of women who get cancer getting it past the age of fifty. Remember those lifestyle choices?

Night-time toilet trips. Yup, up we get at goodness knows what hours.

Seventies

Urinary incontinence. By our seventies, 60% of us will be urinary incontinent. Lovely. There are things we can do, but the Tena Lady pants adverts will suddenly seem less funny (although it is funny that the company insists on using what looks like a thirty-year-old woman in the advert). The reality of incontinence is far from humorous, but it's fine – we're going to crack on and not let it stop us doing anything we want to do. We'll just have to try not to smell of wee, as this isn't a great attribute.

Osteoporosis. One in three of us will have this by now, so again, we're going to be getting on with the yoga/Pilates/balance training, because we don't want a fall, *and* our weight training to help strengthen our bones, aren't we?

Macular degeneration. We can't see fine detail as there are fewer nerve endings sending signals to our brain. Who knew that our eyesight would get worse?

Get yourself to the optician regularly and get some groovy glasses so you don't look like a granny (although you probably will be one by now. At least you can be a groovy granny).

Our **heart** walls are getting thicker and the valves stiffer, but they've still got to pump the same amount of blood so they're all working harder. Exercise and eat a sensible, healthy diet so that you're not clogging up the heart walls further.

Parts of your **brain circuitry** burn out. As late as this? Blimey, I thought mine were gone from forty onwards, but I suspect this means we just become a bit slower.

But it's not all doom and gloom. The massive reward is that many surveys say people's eightieth decade is their happiest decade, for all the good reasons you can imagine. They just accept themselves, finally, as they are.

Let's now go over some of the joys to come in more detail.

Menopause

The menopause is a major feature of midlife and it will affect all of us in different ways. Menopause actually means that a woman's periods have stopped for over twelve months. After that, pretty much everything settles down. No more buying of sanitary products (there's a win right there), our oestrogen levels out and we should begin to feel much better. But before we get to that, we have the perimenopause.

Now, my take on this is not going to be a definitive guide because this isn't a menopause book. What I'm trying to do here is ensure that you've got a grasp on the fact that *anything* can happen during the menopause and whatever's troubling your mind or health might just be menopausal. I will recommend some books by fantastic experts at the back of this one so if you need more help, check them out. But remember, it's important to go and see your doctor if something is worrying you. That's what they are there for.

So, the menopause. There are thirty-four symptoms, allegedly. Lovely.

The best bit is that you don't know when it's going to come upon you. Being pregnant, you can pretty much figure out the date you'll give birth, but with menopause, the range is several years wide. I would advise either going to see your doctor or taking a hormone test (links at the end) which will tell you if your hormones are on the move. The key thing about menopause is that your oestrogen starts diminishing and this can play complete havoc with your system.

Some lucky women have few symptoms and sail through menopause. For others, it is a wretched time of challenges. Most of us sit somewhere in the middle of the spectrum, but how we handle it is totally up to us individually. No one can tell us what's best, no one can challenge our choices. We don't know what will happen, we don't know what choices we'll surprise ourselves by making, but we will all get through it.

Let's look at the possibilities of what might happen during menopause, and don't these read like a bundle of fun?

Brain fog

Lauren Chiren, founder of… how funny is this? I can't remember so I am having to look it up again, #seriousbrainfog. Ah, that's it, www.womenofacertainstage. com. Lauren is an amazing woman who was at the top of her game in the financial world. She then got struck down with dementia, left her job and went home to spend her last few *compos mentis* years with her son. Except she didn't have dementia, it was the menopause.

I spoke to Lauren about this time and she said:

'It was unbelievable, I could not get my head around the fact that I wasn't seriously ill, but that I "just" had the menopause. It had debilitated every aspect of my life and I wasn't going to let that happen to any other women if I could help it. Now I work with employers to raise awareness on menopause and put in place policies for women in peri-menopause."

Lauren's work is hugely important for us all. For example, an employer may design a staff uniform in nylon without a thought for women going through hot flushes, or it may be cut so tight it makes women going through menopause feel flustered and hot, which will place limitations on them. A desk fan may be immensely helpful to midlife female workers. Simple changes could directly affect our performance at work.

Lauren expanded on her work.

'Sometimes, the companies I see have almost a 100% male workforce and the women who are there are under thirty-five, so they [the managers] tell me they've no need to consider the menopause. But I ask them how many of the men [working for the company] have female partners in midlife and don't they consider the impact of the menopause on these men at home? If their partner is having broken sleep, the male workforce may well also be affected by that. In short, the menopause affects us all and it should be looked on as a potential midlife challenge for all of us.'

Heavy periods

Yup, hand up for this one. Heavy periods were my nemesis. Once a month, for several years, I couldn't leave the house at the start of my period because it was so heavy. This meant that I cancelled meetings at short notice because I couldn't travel, I've had to hog toilets on trains, miss flights, take spare black trousers in my handbag along with three to four pairs of pants, and ensure that I had at least four sets of bed linen ready for that time. Just this was enough to make me cry. Utterly humiliating, but completely beyond my control, or so I thought.

Of course, had I been to my GP earlier, I would have found out that there were tablets for this, but I didn't and so suffered for years. If you're suffering with this, get yourself along to your GP. They'll have a whole list of tricks to counteract heavy periods.

Depression

My goodness, this one really isn't funny. I've seen on-line forums where women are talking about ending their lives, they feel so terrible.

It's not surprising some of us get depressed. The shift from who we are to what the menopause makes us into can be startling and a genuine shock to the system. My advice is to get professional help as soon as possible. You cannot do without it and online forums are not the place to seek assistance. It's not fair to ask other women to help you when they probably haven't got the skills. Get real help. Pay for it if you have to, but there are also several charities that specialise in menopausal mental health. Details at the back of this book or on www.toyl.co.uk/pages/the-book

Hot flushes

Known by many of us as the 'Hokey Cokey'. At night, it's 'put your left side in, your left side out, in, out, in, out'… you get the picture. Our favourite question becomes, 'Is it hot in here or is it me?'

Hot flushes are no laughing matter, to be honest. Mine resulted in me wearing shorts and t-shirt throughout winter and as little as possible in summer, while other women spend their lives drenched in sweat. This is mortifying in a meeting where everyone is watching, at night if we need to change the sheets, on the bus… it's horrible and humiliating and I sympathise.

Then of course there are the dreaded night sweats, which are equally horrible. They wake us up, requiring us to either move into a different bed or change the sheets. This can make us think about getting single beds rather than sleeping beside our partner, which is not a way forward.

Insomnia

Yup, we're asleep, asleep, asleep, and then ping! We're completely wide awake. It's 2am. We flick through our phone, but that doesn't help, and then we're still awake. At 7am we're shattered and want to go to sleep, but we can't. It's showtime. Lovely.

Even if you're not plagued by insomnia, you may think, 'I'm definitely getting older as I'm shattered all the time', but actually, in midlife we should be able to do most of the things we could when we were in our twenties. It might not be the menopause, but it could be. Trust me, when I was having heavy periods, I was absolutely shattered and drained. Again, my advice would be to speak to your GP and seek help.

Headaches, anxiety and mood swings

It's not surprising we suffer from headaches as our hormones are on the move. Anxiety can be rather more difficult to cope with. Because it makes us think we are losing our mind, we cannot understand what's happening to us. Bright, confident women can be reduced to housebound messes – of course we're anxious. Again, if this resonates with you, go and see your doctor, check your nutrition and do some exercise to lift your mood with endorphins.

And mood swings? Well, these can just about end any relationship. The challenge is we often don't know we're having them and we're convinced the problem is the other person.

Deep breath, have a think – could it be you? Honestly, this is really tough, but try to be self-aware enough to understand that it may all be down to your mood swings.

Loss of confidence

If I had a pound for every woman who has told me that she's lost confidence in her midlife, I'd be on my own private jet with Brad Pitt one side, mineral water the other, and before you could say, 'Seen much of your ex recently, Brad?' I'd be another forty-five million quid richer.

Here are three of the many quotes I've heard from women about how they feel during menopause:

'I've got such low self-esteem and I don't know what to do about that.'

'I just want to feel better about myself.'

'If I were less anxious it would alleviate my loneliness.'

If this book helps you on any level, I would love it to help you if you've lost your confidence. My goodness, this is just so debilitating for women. For men as well, but we're focusing on us today.

So many things can conspire against us in midlife as it's such a challenge. I'm not a great advocate of prescription drugs, but if you think they can help short term, ask for them. The number-one thing I know will help lift your confidence is exercise. You can even ignore my bit about muscle and bones for now and do any exercise that you enjoy.

Secondly, find someone to talk to, preferably a real person and not an online forum. If you can get professional help, even better, but if not, pick a friend who will genuinely help, not one who's just going to say, 'Me too, babe, let's get the vino out'.

Changes in libido

I've never found anyone who said they wanted more sex during the menopause so this should really read 'loss of libido', but perhaps I'm trying not to scare you too much as the list of symptoms I've included so far isn't much fun.

Oh gosh, here's the thing. You *have* to talk about this one for the sake of your partner (if you have one). If you don't talk, it leads to a downward spiral of loss of intimacy, leading to tension and stress, which adds to your problems in a relationship during the menopause. Please don't misunderstand me, I'm not saying do something you don't want to do at all, but this bit is really hard on partners, so think about the other person in your relationship and see if you can find a way through it. If you're in a relationship then you're in a two-way dialogue, so talk to them about this. Don't just keep saying no; talk about it and find a way forward.

How to help yourself during menopause

Remember the previous chapter on health issues we can control? Reread it. I didn't write it just to fill the pages; I wrote it because everything I recommend points to a reduction in menopause symptoms. If you are a healthy weight, you eat well, you exercise and you've lowered your alcohol and smoking right down (preferably to nil), I know it will have been hard, but it will have been worth it.

Kate Moss has allegedly given up alcohol. What age is she? At the time of writing, she's forty-five. Could it be that she's done it because she is menopausal and knows she has to help herself rather than as a trendy thing to do? It's possible.

There is light at the end of the tunnel. The big plus to menopause is no more period pains, no more sanitary products, no more bloating pre-period, no monthly mood swings and no more leakages. It's absolutely fantastic!

Once you're through to menopause, you really need to ensure that your sex life is back on track, whatever your partner situation. You are too young to give this up, and I think sex is crucial for health. A good friend of mine said, 'I've told my bloke more sex. I don't want my vagina walls collapsing in on themselves.' It's true, they might.

So that's physical health. The reason we have gone into it in so much depth is that our health requirements change in midlife. Our nutritional needs change, our exercise programme changes and our body is changing. Regardless of whether you give two hoots about having a Power Decade or not, every decision you make for your physical health now will impact your old age.

I spoke to Colin Milner, the CEO of the International Council on Active Aging (www.icaa.cc), who is both a friend and an internationally admired expert on active ageing. He said:

'The absolute essential is to live independently for as long as possible. It preserves your quality of life, your savings, your ability to enjoy life. Being independent is the best way to age well and you cannot do this if you haven't looked after yourself physically in the previous decades. The negative effects of living poorly will catch up with us in later life, the exciting part, but by then it's too late.'

If you do care about having your Power Decade, an investment in your physical health will not only mean that you have the energy and stamina to achieve what you want, but will also mean that as you enter the later stages of your life, you will be able to extend your Power Decade (if you want to) and get all the benefits of enjoying an active and independent old age.

Now surely that's something we all want?

4
Your Mental Health

'Create a life that feels good on the inside, not one
that just looks good on the outside.'
—Karen Davis (me), fifty-six, founder of Time of
Your Life

Thank goodness this is a subject that is being taken
so much more seriously these days. When I had a
bout of depression in my twenties, my then husband
advised me not to see a GP because it would be noted
on my medical records and if an employer ever found
out it would go against me. I took his advice as at that
time he was absolutely right. No one admitted mental
health problems as they were not something 'normal'
people got. Goodness knows what treatment anyone
got back in the eighties, if any, because we didn't talk

about it; we 'pulled ourselves together'.

Today, so many people have done work in this area that it's seen in a much broader light, but this book isn't about coping with severe mental health illnesses. You would need professional help for that. It's looking at it in the light of being able to achieve all we want to in our Power Decade.

So, how are you feeling, mentally?

Interestingly, many midlife women I've spoken to lack confidence. They seem fine, go about their daily lives, but when I ask this specific question, it's amazing how many don't believe in themselves.

I went for years giving out self-deprecating comments about my work so as not to appear to be an arrogant little so and so, only to find that after a while I'd started to believe them too. These days, I big up what I do, particularly in business, because otherwise how will people I've just met take me seriously and listen to what I propose? Who will do it for me if I don't do it myself?

Sharron Lowe who is an amazingly inspirational woman, has written a book called *The Mind Makeover*. In this, she talks about how our minds seem to want to tell us negative stuff about ourselves but how women can make the switch to feeling positive about themselves. She writes;

'Hell starts when the person you are now meets the person you could have become. So many women I meet are focusing on negative thoughts. Negative thoughts are like quicksand and you'll sink, pulled down by the things that are wrong or currently lacking in your life.'

In midlife, there are so many things that make women feel negative about themselves, from our changing bodies to society's perception of us once we are forty, the lack of midlife women on TV (women over fifty-five watch more TV than any other group yet there are precious few women over fifty on TV compared to men over fifty) and the attitude of some of us who are mentally on a countdown to retirement. But we are intelligent women. We know exactly how much we have achieved to get us and our loved ones this far. We know exactly how many skills we've needed, how much juggling we've had to do and how much work we've put in to make everyone's life around us amazing. We know the incredible challenges we've faced, which seemed insurmountable at the time, but surprise! We did get through them. It's time to genuinely believe that we can do what we want to do.

Be mindful

Mental self-sabotage is the greatest harm we do ourselves. We can achieve anything, yet we tell ourselves all sorts of negative stuff. There's a reason I've only got around to writing this book at fifty-six, and that's because I wasn't sure I was good enough to write. Secondly, I was always working to push others forward in their achievements. Family or clients, it was never my turn as all my energies had to be put into other people's stories. I let that happen.

Don't be hard on yourself. Let's move your mindset to where you're going to put yourself right up there, in first place, because without you being on top form, how can you help others?

The brilliance of today's world is that there are so many ways to talk yourself into achievement, and a great place to start is with a mind-calming app on your phone. I've got Buddhify, but there is Calm, the Mindfulness App, Headspace – so many. Do a bit of research and find one you like. Of course, you must then use it. Every day. Most of the successful women I know spend around ten minutes a day working on mindfulness, calming themselves and focusing on what they need to do. Mindfulness is the easiest way to calm your inner voice, but if this isn't going to work for you, there are a couple of books I'd recommend which you'll find in the resources list at the end.

Be fabulous

Many women love the beauty industry. It makes us feel great. People are behind the beauty store counters, working to make us look (and feel) amazing. Yes, they want to sell us stuff, but we are likely to be more than happy to buy it if it boosts our confidence, and that is what the beauty industry is all about: confidence.

I'm going to talk about beauty because confidence is tied up closely with our mental health, but we often forget that we are now older than we were when we created our makeup and skincare routine. We need to revisit it to ensure that we are looking our best, so I'm also going to look at cosmetic procedures.

Beauty

'I personally don't think people look better when they do it [have cosmetic surgery]; they just look different... And if you're doing it out of fear, that fear's still going to be seen through your eyes.'
—Cate Blanchett, forty-nine, actress

Now if I had Cate Blanchett's bone structure, I'd probably say the same, but let's not be too quick to judge others, eh, Cate? I'm just going to point out the options.

I love beauty products, the promises, the possible transformations and the confidence that they have given to millions of women from the dawn of time. It's an industry like no other, totally bound up with our psyche.

Midlife is a time to relearn makeup and skincare, because what we've been doing all these years needs to be reimagined for midlife. I'm in no way saying become more conservative in your makeup, but if you haven't had professional help with it in the last five years, make an appointment at the counter of a brand you like and see what's changed since you last looked. First, going to a makeup counter makes you feel great. It's pure self-care, so do it. Second, you will learn something new. It could be a way to apply a colour or a look, but you will definitely learn something great. Thirdly, if you've used the same products for years, how do you know what's out there? Beauty is a massively innovative industry and new products, colours and looks are coming out all the time, and some of these will be perfect for you.

Makeup counters are amazing places these days. Usually you pay between £30–£50 to have a makeover and it's deducted from the cost of any products you buy. The makeup expert really needs you to end up looking great because they want to sell product, so you're likely to come out feeling pretty good. Don't dismiss anything they do that you haven't done before, like cat flicks or lashes, even if your natural reaction is to dismiss it as 'not you'. You haven't seen it on you before.

Take the look home, live with it for an afternoon and see if you can get used to it. Don't make instant decisions. What we're trying to avoid is being stuck in our ways. It's incredibly easy to go through midlife wearing the same makeup look we wore in our twenties or thirties, but this won't do. Midlife is a key time for self-care, so if beauty is important to you, keep your look current. Reimagine yourself every five years or you could look dated.

Lee Pycroft is a makeup artist who has had her hands on the faces of Elle Macpherson, Anne Hathaway and Joely Richardson. In recent years, Lee retrained as a Human Givens psychotherapist and she now works in both industries. What makes Lee so interesting is that she has also won a hero award from Help for Heroes for her charity work (she also understands the value of volunteering) where she uses beauty as self-care to boost wellbeing in the vulnerable sectors of society, because she understands the connection between beauty, confidence and mental health. It's an incredible subject that Lee dedicates her www. pocketsofwisdom.co.uk videos to, so take a look if you get a moment.

I talked to Lee about the changing face of beauty for midlife women and here are her top tips:

'You've got to start with your skin. If that's glowing and vibrant, half the job is done. Once you've done that, look at your brows and get them shaped. They are likely to thin as you get older, so consider brow dyes, powder or pencils to redefine them every day. You'll be amazed at what a difference defined brows make to your face. Likewise, lashes – these can also thin or lighten as you enter midlife, so think about getting up to speed with applying these [false eyelashes] as they lighten up your face and these days they absolutely don't make you look like a pantomime dame!'

Lee is a great believer in tinted moisturiser with sun protection factor (SPF).

'Sun damage is very real so apply SPF every day. Sun is essential for our health, but keep your face out of it at all times. There are so many great products with SPF in them with a bit of colour that you just don't need natural sunlight on your face. Couple this with a soft liquid blusher, use a lip pencil to define thinning lips before gloss or lipstick and you've got your basic look ready.'

Revisit your skincare routine in midlife along with your makeup, because your needs will change. Over-the-counter stuff may not be enough, and if you're really interested get a dermatologist on your side.

Cosmetic surgery

I talked to award-winning dermatologist Dr Vicky Dondos of www.medicetics.com about what happens to facial structure in midlife. Vicky is an incredibly well-known expert in subtle anti-ageing medicine. To you and me, this means injectables, lasers, facials and skincare treatments that are more medical than natural. I love her work as she is kind and plays for subtlety rather than major change.

'Face structure changes as you age and some of the biggest changes are in the eye socket and jawline. The eye socket skin drops so that the tear duct creates a hollow under the eye – bags, if you like. The skin here is very thin so this can emphasise dark rings or the hollow. At the same time, jowl lines can become more pronounced and lines start to shape the face more than in earlier years. It's just a question of managing these.'

Vicky tells me there's a lot we can do, but things like jowls are likely to need surgery if you're really that committed. It all depends on your perspective. Personally, surgery is a bit too far for me, but many mates have had their eyes done. It's up to them as they're the ones who live with it. Just be clear as to why you are doing anything. If it is for confidence, be sure it's about the physical issue and not something else.

Look at Jane Fonda as an example. At eighty-one years old, Jane has been candid that she felt her cosmetic surgery four years ago gave her career a further ten years. She's also been frank about having started messing around with her face due to the desire to create a 'mask' – a front for the world – because of sexual abuse at an early age.

> 'On one level, I hate the fact that I've had the need to alter myself physically to feel that I'm OK.'
> —Jane Fonda

Jane's a powerful, strong, opinionated woman, and yet she talked herself into surgery through insecurities in her head. Insecurity can get to us all, so don't judge yourself too harshly; just be honest about your reasons if you're considering surgery. What do you think it will solve for you?

I was at a conference late last year where a gorgeous woman, a multi-millionaire who has advised No 10 Downing Street and is an MBE, was talking about her business. She made a comment about how she'd been on the BBC news talking about XYZ, stating that the best thing about it was that the BBC hair and makeup artists made her look ten years younger.

OMG, what chance do we stand if such an accomplished, confident, poised woman (and she was fantastic) thinks that looking ten years younger is so important? What chance have midlife women got of owning their age, being proud of their immense achievements and standing tall if even the sisterhood is buying a 'youth is best' mantra? Physical ageing is *not* something we should be ashamed of.

I pulled the speaker up on her comments – nicely, when she was on her own – and said as much to her. She really thought about what I'd said and was genuinely shocked at how easily her comment had come to her. She then relayed a story about a female colleague of hers, a director on a major corporate board, who had nearly died on the operating table having a face-lift as she felt her fellow (male) directors were judging her for her age. Even worse, after recovery, she went back for more surgery.

The interesting thing is that this woman's story, just like Jane Fonda's, was prefaced by 'I felt'. No man had said directly to her that her older face was stopping her doing business. No one said to Jane that her mature look was stopping her getting acting roles, it's just what the women 'felt'.

Why do we feel this? Why do we not think, 'Ooh, maybe I need a different business offering. Maybe the board just doesn't like what I say'? We have to stop self-sabotaging.

Eat well, exercise, take care of yourself, go out into the world, but never be ashamed of how you look. Midlife women are the fastest growing demographic in the world, and the quicker the rest of the world gets that, the sooner older women will stop changing themselves surgically because we will be the norm.

My final advice to you if you're considering surgery is don't make your decision based on price. You'll regret it – you'll quite possibly be a source of gossip for your friends for a while, but not in a good way. Bad injectables and surgery are very noticeable – just look at certain celebrities.

Hair

We can get really stuck in our ways with hair and assume that what worked for us at thirty will see us through into midlife. It won't. As with makeup, that just won't do.

My hairdresser, Jon Moore, trained with Trevor Sorbie before striking out on his own as a hair consultant, and now he advises women of all ages on the styles that look best for them as well as looking after their hair in their homes. Whenever I've got an event coming up, he's the one I call to blow dry me to boost my confidence on the day.

Jon and I discussed hair in midlife and he agreed that it's got to be seen in its own right.

'The worst thing I see on midlife women is long, dark hair; it just isn't flattering. For me, length should never be longer than the collar bone as it just drags the face and any style down. Shorter hair can keep it's bounce and frame the face so much better.'

Jon also says that the texture of hair changes.

'As you get older, you can totally see the effects of lower oestrogen levels. Hair is duller, coarser and thinner, and I can always tell if a client is on hormone replacement treatment (HRT) as their hair is like a twenty-year-old's. However, HRT has its problems, so you've just got to weigh up what you want. Likewise, grey hair is coarser than your hair used to be and you have to be careful not to heat treat it too much as it will just break. Serum it into control if it's not doing what you want it to do.'

We also discussed short hairstyles on midlife women.

'It's got to have a bit of movement, shine and colour, even if that colour is grey. There's no problem with grey, but if your hair is like a helmet, without texture and movement, it's just not going to be an asset that is working hard for you. Go to your hairdresser and have a really good chat about new styles because it's worth experimenting and trying something new.'

Speaking of grey hair, remember those lines of ladies in salons all getting their purple rinses once their hair had gone grey? Well, in midlife it comes to us all. Not necessarily the purple rinse, although many of us do seem to be going for pink these days, but the choice of whether to embrace grey or deny it the light of day and keep going with the full-on colour is one that we all face.

I'm lucky enough to have the multi-award-winning salon owned by Chris Williams, who is International Colour Director at Rush, local to me. He's been my co-lourist for years, so on my latest visit we chatted about midlife hair.

'I would absolutely tell a woman not to go to grey, but then you might think I would because of my job. Not so. Think about it: your hair surrounds your face and the colour of your hair will reflect into your skin. If you have warm golden tones in your hair, your skin looks healthy, but if your skin is reflecting off grey hair then it's going to look washed out and sallow. If you go for grey, rethink your makeup so that you can bump up the warmth to counter-act this.'

What about if we go platinum?

'Well, that doesn't suit everyone, but again, rethink your makeup. White is pretty unforgiving so be sure before you do it. Remember all hair in midlife needs a bonding product to help smooth it, but otherwise choose colour or not and remember to rethink your makeup.'

So what were the purple rinses (I actually saw one recently) that midlife ladies seemed to love in our youth all about?

'Funnily enough, purple rinses were an accidental thing. The setting lotions used in the seventies to create and hold styles with rollers used to get into grey hair and, over time, the hair took on the purple colour. Women then thought it was a thing so started asking for it at their salon. These days, colour can be much wilder with women asking for all sorts, but warm colours always look best with skin.'

What about roots?

'There are loads of touch-up products to get you through to your next appointment without having grey roots give you away. L'Oréal does a great range of aerosols, but there are many powders as well. Just pick something darker than your colour as dark roots will look better than lighter roots.'

So, there you have it from one of the UK's top colourists. If you're in or around Chichester in West Sussex, do go and see him; he's one of the most chilled men I know, a top hair colourist, and employing the help of an expert is essential to achieving a great look.

Now let's unpack what the supermodels and celebrities advise us from their Instagram pages. Juice diets, vegan diets, air diets – goodness, they do spout a lot of stuff at us, don't they? No question, many of them look utterly amazing, so let's delve a little deeper, shall we?

Celebrities look fantastic and ooze confidence

Yes, they do, but supermodels get to be supermodels because they look extraordinary in the first place. They have something the rest of us don't; they are freaks of nature: beautiful, gorgeous, stunning, but rare. That's why they are valued, because they are not like the rest of us.

Most of us are, by definition, average. Nothing wrong with that, them's the breaks, but we cannot be super-models because of genetics and whatever we were dealt at birth, so let's give that dream up. What super-models do to look great hasn't got much relevance to us mere mortals. We don't have the chefs, the trainers, the support teams that they do because we are, well, mere mortals.

But we can learn from them, so what advice should we take from celebs?

Drink lots of water. This is jolly good stuff and 2 litres of it a day will do you only good.

Avoid sugar. This is not good stuff so don't eat much of it. (Fruit as well should be limited.)

Avoid alcohol. Many celebs don't touch the stuff because it's empty calories, it's not great for their energy levels when their schedules are stuffed full, and it's a physically ageing product. Give it up (or mostly, except for high days and holidays).

Get enough sleep. Yup, sleep is good, but not too much. Eight hours is lovely, but no more. If you're struggling with insomnia, and many of us are, then it's worth going to see your doctor. There are over-the-counter remedies, but also the app you may have downloaded for mindfulness probably has sleep programmes on it. Mine has six 'go to sleep' meditations as well as six 'can't sleep' ones. I also use a 'sleep spray' for pillows, usually lavender based and a hot bath with something like Aromatherapy Associates Deep Relax bath oil can be amazing.

Go vegan. There's no question that a more plant-based diet is a good thing, but don't forget that celebs may well have chefs balancing their diets correctly for them. If you want to be vegan, take it seriously and ensure that your diet is balanced so that you are getting all the vitamins, minerals and nutrition that you need.

It's easy to have an unbalanced diet as a vegan, so take care of yourself. Really, I'd just suggest going towards more plant-based meals where you lay off the cheese a bit as well (it's the high fat content, not the dairy that's the challenge with cheese).

Juicing. I know some people swear by this, but I can't see it as a permanent way forward. Do it for a bit, focusing on veg rather than fruit, but ultimately, we're not meant to juice full time. It'll muck up our digestive systems long term.

Go carbohydrate free. I see this a lot with celebs: 'Ooh, no carbs, no carbs', but I think this is a nuanced rule and what they are actually trying to do is cut down on white carbs, such as white bread, white rice and white pasta. Many foods have carbs in them, from carrots to spinach, so these celebs don't mean no carbs at all.

Me, I'm all for a bit of moderation. I definitely eat carbs such as hummus and veggies, but I try to avoid the white ones, purely because of the calories. I can't afford them without two hours of spinning attached to their consumption, but you cannot tell me that a plate of chips is not one of the most fantastic joys in life. Even Meghan Markle is said to indulge on her birthday, which helps prove that the combination of fat and carbs is one of the greatest culinary delights ever. So it's a yes to carbs, but have a think about the ones you want to eat.

Stop smoking. Lots of celebs smoke, but we won't see a photo of them doing so, it's bad PR. They smoke for all the reasons that any of us do: appetite suppressant, stress relief, more stress relief, and because they enjoy it. But smoking is bad for us, our skin and health, so it's not something for midlife. Celebs and supermodels have makeup artists to cover up the damage to their skin, we don't. Give it up. Sorry...

Exercise. Almost every celebrity will have a personal trainer, even those who hate exercising. Looking good is their currency so when they post photos of themselves exercising, they really are doing it. Not only that, they are pushing themselves way harder in their sessions than you or I would. When they deny exercising at all and claim that they're naturally fit from 'running around all day', raise an eyebrow.

The benefits of exercise to celebs are they have more energy to get through their gruelling days, they look better when papped, they can get into the size zero loan frocks they get offered and there's more of a glow in their skin as a starting point for any photo shoot. We are not celebrities so we don't need to work as hard, depending on how we want to look, but exercise is a good thing for us all with huge benefits, so let's get this into our daily routine.

Weird beauty treatments. Vampire facials, ruby facials, $2 million humidifiers, placenta facials, Evian baths – gosh, it's exhausting trying to keep up. But here's the thing, why are we being told about these outrageous treatments? Is it so we will want to try them or is it to get coverage in the press for the celebrity?

Here's how I think it goes down. A-lister celeb is at the top of their game, but fear is ever present. There is always someone newer and hotter coming along on their heels, which means that their fan base, endorsements and opportunities could be taken away from them, so they try some of the more outrageous treatments to drink longer from the Fountain of Youth as they believe it will extend their careers. They also get further press coverage because the treatments are so extraordinary, keeping them in the public eye, and in the eye of companies that endorse them or film producers who might feature them.

Are these weird and wonderful treatments for you and me? If you have extraordinary amounts of cash and fancy it, why not? Just remember you will get more benefits from your diet, mental health, skincare and exercise regimes.

Injectables and surgery. Kylie Jenner's effect on lip injectables was incredible, wasn't it? Absolutely unbelievable that overnight everyone wanted to have bee-stung lips and she's made a $900 million fortune from it. It didn't happen when Bridget Bardot first appeared, nor when Emmanuelle Béart looked so stunning in *Manon des Source*, but it did with Kylie Jenner.

Kylie reportedly had her lips done because she was on one of her first ever dates with a bloke she liked and he said, 'I didn't think you would be a good kisser because you have such small lips.' As a young girl, Kylie found that difficult to take, which is sad, even with a $900 million fortune off the back of it.

If you're going to have any kind of cosmetic surgery, don't do it for others, do it for you.

Now we know what we need to do to get ourselves in top shape for midlife. Yes, it is an effort, but ask yourself if you really want to contemplate the alternatives?

- Going into old age in poor physical shape, dogged by illness and lack of mobility
- Not becoming the person you believe you could be
- Living midlife as a waiting room for retirement
- Accepting that adventures are not on the midlife agenda
- Regret

As Sharron Lowe says, the hell of you now meeting the you that you could have become is almost too awful to contemplate. We are running out of time, but we can have our Power Decade and be that better version of ourselves. It's still all there for the taking, there is still time, but now is your moment. Take it.

5

The Time Of Your Life Methodology

'I've discovered that this is your moment to reinvent yourself after years of focusing on the needs of everyone else.'
—Oprah Winfrey

And that is the most fantastic, brilliant thing about the Power Decade: it will all be yours. But first, what is a Power Decade?

In short, it's a ten-year action plan that we make once we've done an audit of where we are and what we want to achieve. We're going to take stock and weigh each aspect of our lives against how important it is to us, then we're going to create one-, five- and ten-year goal sets so that we can achieve them.

Simple.

To help you with your Power Decade plan, I've come up with the Time of Your Life (TOYL) method. It goes like this.

T is for taupe

I bet you weren't expecting that, eh?

Taupe. Describe it. Grey with a tinge of brown.

Do you know what? That's what midlife women have allowed themselves to become too often. Taupe (it could also describe my hair.) Kelly Hoppen (celebrity interior designer) loves it. Give her a bit of taupe and she'll be off down Vicky Beckham's Cotswold pile with a decorating swatch before you can say 'Zen's the job'.

Why does she love taupe? Here's what she says:

> 'Taupe is calm, quiet, and very easy to live with. It is not overbearing and it does not shout out and demand attention. For this reason, taupe is ideal to use in instilling a sense of calm into a room. It is the perfect colour to provide a

remedy to the stressful pace of frenetic modern life.'

And doesn't that describe the midlife woman down to a tee?

We provide an incredibly calming backdrop for everyone else in our lives as they add the colourful highlights to the taupe we've created. We're there for everyone, soothing arguments, providing flat deposits, cooking meals for all, sending cash up to students, checking on ageing parents, getting work done, putting out for partners – it's incessant, this twirling of everything to make it all happen so that the lives around us can carry on.

But what about us? What is there for us except more taupe? Where are our flashes of light, our silvers, golds and cerises set against this taupe?

Let's go back. We midlife women make 67% of all buying decisions in the UK, but 88% of women over fifty don't think advertisers are interested in talking to us. 'Commercially stale' is a phrase I've heard used about us. We are the fastest growing demographic worldwide, and yet we believe brands are ignoring us. Why? Because we are letting them, because we don't kick up.

Taupe.

Now I'm not saying that we need to get our Action Girl pants on and become overtly political, but if we want some of our own colours to come out in midlife, if we don't just want to be the taupe background makers, we're going to have to start getting a bit active and exerting our power, which is real. Do we want our midlife to pass us by as being a time when we enabled things to happen for everyone else while our own dreams were sidelined because we were done in and had nothing left for us?

We are incredibly good at being self-sacrificing. We love our families, whatever their makeup, and we are really good at easing their way through the years. We are unbelievable at this.

But…

We don't come this way again, and do you know what? We're not doing anyone a favour by easing their way so completely; it will only lead to us being unfulfilled and out of energy for what *we* want to do. We need to have our Power Decade when we can really get into what we want to do for ourselves, and by gosh we're going to have it. Now that's exciting.

Let's be honest, we are going to have to keep on with the taupe to a certain extent, but we are going to push further. We are going to do stuff that excites us, we are going to make a change. We are going to be selfish!

I realise at this point that some of you will be uneasy. You have put everyone else first for so long that this will be a struggle, but trust me, it is going to make your life fantastic. You are not going to be invisible as a midlife woman, you are not going to feel ignored by advertisers and society; you are going to be trail-blazing, my girl, and loving every single minute of it because you'll be doing it with others, both like you and different to you. You are going to be respected in your community as a woman full of life and wisdom, a women of fun, a woman whose opinion will be sought out and her views listened to. You are no longer going to be seen as just someone's mother, someone's part-ner, someone's daughter; you are going to be talked about with awe and love. Now, doesn't that sound more like it than sitting at home, watching TV, wait-ing for friends or family to get in touch or a humdrum job to end in retirement?

I read somewhere that no one makes new friends after forty. What utter tosh. You, my lovely, are about to em-bark on the adventure of your life. This is not a midlife crisis; it's an adventure where we, en masse, start mo-bilising for the good of our community, families and friends. *We* are the difference in this new world – how exciting is that?

We are going to have fun! Even better, we are going to make a difference to this world between us and we do that with O and Y. But remember, T is for selfish. I know that doesn't really make sense, but taupe is set to remind you not to be this, not to revert to your default position.

By the way, don't blame Kelly Hoppen for the taupe thing. I love her interiors and hope you do too. She's a hard-working bird, but she just made a statement about taupe that was too good not to use. Big hugs, Kels…

O is for others

'As you grow older, you will discover that you have two hands, one for helping yourself, the other for helping others.'
—Audrey Hepburn, 1929–1993, actress

OK, you've spent your life so far looking after others at home, at work, more people at home, friends – you're exhausted from looking after others. That's not what I'm talking about here.

I've spent a bit of time in the USA in the last few years and we have nothing on the Americans in terms of a culture of volunteering. I'm not saying that their society is better than ours, but their whole culture is geared towards volunteering. 'Giving back', if you like.

For example, during freshers' week, college students are taken, en masse, into local community projects and assigned a day's work as a gesture of goodwill and service to their new hometown. Our students just seem to get legless and make work for the local community with various high jinks involving the relocation of traffic cones and bodily fluid deposits that will then need to be washed down. Now I'm not saying that UK students shouldn't have a good time, but I'm sure you can see the immediate difference in outlook. In this country, we understand volunteering almost in terms of 'community service', ie it's a punishment for us having been naughty.

Why do we see it as a bad thing and not a good thing? I assume it's because we're pretty tired after a day's work. We're wrestling with the menopause, and now I've asked you to chuck in regular exercise, eating well and getting eight hours' sleep, so I'm not leaving you masses of time. But I want you to consider volunteering for something completely new, too.

Make it something that you think you might like because your superpower is about to come alive here.

I read this week that there are five different triggers that make midlife women press the 'activate' button to focus on real change in our lives:

- **Illness**. This probably means serious illness rather than a cold; the type of illness that makes you understand the fragility of life and push for major change in your health or how you live.

- **Injustice**. How far this one motivates you into action depends on how much it touches your soul and your anger. You might be unhappy about the plight of refugees, but do you give a bit of cash or actually do something?

- **Disadvantage**. This motivates many of us to beat the odds. Apparently, equal pay for women is expected in 217 years from now, despite UK equal pay legislation being passed in 1970 – does this anger you and get you motivated?

- **Inequality.** This gets me motivated. I see lots of groups getting their voices heard, but the midlife woman, the fastest growing demographic on this planet, is discriminated against all the time.

- **Underprivileged**. Does this get you going? All those people who are perfectly able but haven't had the advantages of birth/money/contacts to get ahead?

In truth, all of these could motivate us into action, but quite often we doubt ourselves. We shouldn't. I believe midlife women are the most skilful, brave, resourceful, amazing sector of society there is, but we just don't get involved enough in creating change.

What about looking at ways you can change the world around you? For me, volunteering is a fantastic way to do this. Nobody can sack me, I can pick my hours and I can say exactly what I think as there's no chance of a disciplinary hearing. But more importantly, I can work for change, for good. Have a think. In my opinion, you can do more good in this world as a midlife woman than anyone else out there because you've dealt with so much and you're still standing.

We midlife women start with others because that's just the way we roll. We are going to show our communities how we can all make a difference while Instagrammers are showing us sunsets and their perfect thong-clad arses around the world. We will each strive for small gains until the collective whole of our work makes an impact that will resonate even unto the United Nations. I'm not kidding, I'm deadly serious.

Here's what I suggest we do and how we're going to do it.

The United Nations has seventeen Sustainable Development Goals to help all of humanity. These were created in 2015 by people far brighter than me, but even I can see how they make sense. You can find these objectives online at www.globalgoals.org

These goals need to be achieved by 2030, which doesn't give us much time. No one asked us midlife women, the fastest growing demographic, what we wanted, but we're going to let that go at present. No time for a strop here.

Have a look at the seventeen goals and see which one appeals to you. Pick any one; I'm sure there are enough for something to appeal to you. One of my sons is involved in clean water as he says that everything else is secondary to having access to water. For me, it's about making communities inclusive, and for my husband it's all about good health and wellbeing.

When you have chosen your goal, give your time, not cash, to it, and there's a reason for this. The entire point is for us to engage in the wider world, to mobilise ourselves as a force for good. Cash means that someone else is making decisions for us while we're sitting on the sofa, watching the world go by on a TV screen where midlife women are woefully absent. I want *you* to make decisions about social issues in the world because you've got the experience and knowledge to do so. Also, as you're doing it unpaid, there is *no* agenda against the decisions you make.

Let's start using the worksheets in this book. These can be found in the Worksheets section at the back of the book or downloaded from my website at www.toyl.co.uk/pages/the-book

These are for you, they're private, they're your thoughts, so write down whatever appeals to you.

At the top of the Volunteer Sheet, write down how many hours you think you can find a week or month to give as a volunteer. I'd suggest a minimum of four hours, which is one hour per week. That's fifty-two hours in a year, which is just over two days. I've probably spent longer on Candy Crush in past years, so it's perfectly doable. Start with four hours per month and see what happens.

OK, now note down what skills you can offer or what you'd like to try. Think about what might interest you and make a note on the sheet.

If we take me, for example, I'm interested in the stats that say 50% of us in 2017 (there are no newer stats at the time of writing), regardless of age or gender, were lonely for a significant amount of time. I'm sure that's worse for younger and older people, but it affects all of us, so I want to have a socially inclusive community in my village that actively cares for all residents of all ages.

Next.

So what now? We're sitting on the sofa with our ideological mission in mind, we've allocated time, but we're still sitting on the sofa. How do we make this happen?

Well, this is the fun bit.

> 'Your job is for living, giving to others is to live life.'
> —Ricky Gervais, *Derek*, episode 4

If we want to do this, we're going to have to make it work ourselves. How? We're going to get up off the sofa, go to the internet and do a bit of trawling.

Before you start, ponder how wide you want your involvement to be. Do you want to dip in and out of different projects around the country or do you want one project really close to home that you can stay with long term? Personally, I'm not going to go for anything too big or too far from home as there's only so much I can do, so I'm going to do something for my village and not try to be bigger or cleverer than that, but this is just my version. Make a note in 'Others' as to where you want your work to count.

There are volunteering holidays, weekends and all sorts of choices out there. What appeals to you? Some chap recently got an OBE for giving all his holidays to volunteering on the Cornish Coast, repairing fences and so on, so it's perfectly doable, but whatever it is, you need to leave your home to do it.

This is key. You need to go into the big, wide world and call it an adventure. You need to meet people of all ages you wouldn't normally find in everyday life, and you need to meet them in person, not virtually. My volunteering has brought me into working contact with a ninety-year-old and a seventeen-year-old, which is a key objective for me and my understanding of the world. I get to see issues from young and old eyes and it affects my fixed views of life in a brilliant, vibrant, challenging way.

But why are we even bothering? Because there are so many benefits to doing this, I'm only going to list a few of them.

One, how often do we moan at others to get off their personal screens? If we don't get off our own phones or iPads and do something meaningful in the world, how can we ever expect anyone else, such as children and grandchildren, to follow our example and do the same? How will they understand the benefits unless we can tell them the stories about what we have got up to, inspiring them with the difference we've made? Most people under the age of twenty genuinely feel a responsibility to our planet, so why don't we show them how to activate that feeling for good?

Two, research by the *British Medical Journal* (no less) into the benefits of mental wellbeing and volunteering found 'The association between volunteering and wellbeing did not emerge during early adulthood to mid-adulthood, instead becoming apparent above the age of 40 years and continuing up to old age'. In other words, if you volunteer after the age of forty, there are real and tangible benefits for your mental wellbeing. Lovely.

Three, the liberation of unpaid work is something to experience. This really surprised me. With unpaid work, I'm there because it's something I want to make a difference at, but if someone suggests a meet that I think is pointless, I don't have to go and no one can fire me. I can suggest things without fear of ridicule and loss of status. I can reinvent myself as the person I really am at my core rather than what I may have

THE TIME OF YOUR LIFE METHODOLOGY

become in corporate life. I can truthfully say if I don't agree with someone's idea – nicely, obvs – and can disagree with minimal consequences. This impacts on how I feel about voluntary work and flows through into my day job in a great way.

Four, your current friends are probably all around the same age as you. This is not healthy in mid and later life. Your ideas and influences are fixed into a demographic that is like you. Volunteering cuts through this and exposes you to a whole load of influences that you might never have come into contact with. Embrace them all, let them challenge your current thinking. Getting younger and older views into your life is a fine thing.

Also, given that your friends are likely all the same age as you, you will age together. Friends will pass and your social circle will narrow. Volunteering means that you will instantly make new friends, which is a good thing for widening your friendship circles.

Five, volunteering brings you into contact with all of humanity. Use this as an opportunity to look at the kind of later-life person you want to be. You'll see them all. The moaners, the ones with a tiny life, the generous, the wise, the active, the infirm. Take a long, hard look at all of the older people you encounter and decide who you want to be as you age.

Then look the other way and see what you can learn from the younger generation of volunteers you work with. What are their dreams and hopes? Can you help them on their way with advice? See how their vision might impact yours.

Jonty, fifty-one, works every week for Riding for the Disabled. I asked her why she did it?

Her answer was to send me to have a look at the YouTube video about Angelika Trabert, an equestrian and winner of twenty-four medals, six of them at five different Paralympic games. Jonty pointed me to the key quote from this amazing woman: 'If I sit on the horse and if the horse really understands me, I'm just free'. In other words, she's free in a way she can never be in a wheelchair. And that's it. Jonty does her voluntary work from a kind corner of her heart because she is also a rider and knows what it's like to have the freedom and understanding of a horse. Animals don't judge and Jonty wants that freedom and non-judgment for those with disabilities.

Six, helping others has been a fundamental trait of being human since the dawn of time, but many of us have forgotten this. I cannot tell you enough how volunteering has impacted my life for the better. It has given me lifelong friends, so many great laughs, a new understanding of the needs of different generations, confidence in my abilities, challenges that stretch my abilities and tolerance levels, plus work that has made a real difference to my community. Make it an essential part of your midlife. Try different things, embrace what you get out of it and be amazed at what you find you can give.

If 10,000 people read this book and half of you decide to give one hour per week to volunteering in the next year, that's over 250,000 hours, 31,250 working days, 6,250 working weeks or the work of 120 full-time employees going back into our communities. This is your superpower, so unleash it on the world and see how amazingly bright it shines. You will likely blow yourself away with what a brilliant force for good you are. Even now, I cannot believe the difference I've made in some tiny way to people's lives. Now that's job satisfaction, and on just four hours per month. It's incredible. What are you waiting for?

We are working to find good mental health, a positive place in our heads so that we can ace our Power Decade. Volunteering is absolutely not a distraction from our Power Decade; it is great for mental health. Start small if you're not sure, start your own charity if you are. Volunteering has no downside for either you or the recipient and it will improve your wellbeing.

Y is for you

> 'The most important relationship you have in life is the one you have with yourself.'
> —Diane von Fürstenberg, seventy-two, designer

It took me a long time to understand this, but it is true. The root of our happiness in all our relationships with others starts with whether we are happy with ourselves.

Getting into a good relationship with ourselves is tricky. We know ourselves intimately, but we can't always control what we do. We are rarely proud of ourselves or give ourselves any credit for anything, we often don't like how we look and we are immensely self-critical. In fact, if a friend of ours thought about us like we think of ourselves, we probably wouldn't be friends.

Why do we do this to ourselves? Life is hard enough without us beating ourselves up on a regular basis. Honestly, that little voice in our head that gives space to negative dialogue really does have a lot to answer for.

See this bit as couples' therapy. You and that little voice are going to be working out how to improve your relationship because you need to be comfortable with you. You don't need some part of you telling you that you're not good enough at whatever it's on about that day; you need a little voice in your head cheerleading for you, being kind to you, willing you to win and finding ways for you to do so every moment possible. You deserve it, you've worked for it, and by golly, we're going to get it for you.

There are so many great books out there on how to get the little voice in your head to talk positively to you, and these could be a good place to start. *The Chimp Paradox* by Professor Steve Peters is one and previously mentioned *The Mind Makeover* by Sharron Lowe is another, but there are more at the back of this book. If your inner voice is really negative, seek professional help. Being at peace with ourselves is not something we can leave until our seventies (that's when the stats say we finally get a grip on this).

Your relationships with your partner, friends, parents and children are all functions of how you feel about yourself. If you bitch about your friends behind their backs, it's likely that you're unhappy with yourself. If you're picking on your partner all the time, it's likely that you're unhappy with yourself. If you're clinging to your children as they forge their way in the world and are bereft at their leaving home, it's likely that you're unhappy with yourself. All your relationships start with you, because if you're at peace with yourself, you're not always thinking about how you feel, giving you time to open up and see how others feel and what you can do for them.

The reason I wrote this book is that so many women have got to midlife and feel unhappy with how their lives have turned out. Well, guess what: our partners may well feel the same. For our Power Decade, we are going to lift our vision from our navels and see how we can help others.

Do you really think life has turned out exactly how the midlife men you know thought it would? Do you think they don't have broken dreams and frustrations? Unlike women, the first question men will be asked in most new social situations is 'What do you do for a living?' Nothing about if they are kind, decent people; for men, it's all about being alpha, which generally relates to what they have achieved in terms of finance or status. How draining must that be? A whole life taken down to money and a job title. Now, this book isn't about men's challenges, it's about ours, but to have great relationships with the men in our lives, shouldn't we stop judging them and work to help them by being kind?

Work to lift your vision from you to how others feel. If someone's not so nice to you, it's really not an issue. Not everyone is going to like you, think like you or react like you, so let it go. Be kind. This is one of the greatest gifts you can give yourself and your relationships during your Power Decade.

L is for living

> 'Ageing isn't about getting old, it's about LIVING.'
> —Cameron Diaz, forty-six, actress

And that's right at the heart of what this book is about. Living. Midlife is for living and living brilliantly.

Of course, challenges are going to arise, which is why you need to be in the best of physical and mental health so that you can cope with them, but living well is the greatest reward you can have.

Do you remember when I said that we may well have got stuck in a makeup routine from our twenties? It's the same with living. Kids or no kids, most of us hit midlife doing exactly the same as we did in our twenties and thirties, but that's not living. That's not extending our repertoire. Think about how much technology has changed our lives in the past ten years – has your life fundamentally altered during that time?

We have so many more options now than we did ten years ago and we need to go out, find them and evolve, or become stuck in our ways, irrelevant to the next generation coming through (which will include our grandchildren, if we have any). Our Power Decade is all about extending our range and being careful about where we spend our time, because that's all we've really got. Time is the greatest leveller in the world as we all have the same twenty-four hours each day to engage with life.

What are you going to do with those twenty-four hours?

Let's start at home.

Let's start with you.

6
The Power Decade Plan

'The big secret in life is that there is no secret.
Whatever your goal, you can get there if you're
willing to work.'
—Oprah Winfrey

I'm going to assume that you've taken my advice and
got yourself healthy and fit, and possibly spent quite
a long time on it, so let's get some positive aspects of
the Power Decade on the go.

We're going to start with you by making our Power
Decade list, splitting it into sections. We can put anything we want on it, no limit, but we need to be sure
we *really* want to do it because we are going to make
it happen. The Power Decade worksheet is at the back

of the book and you can download it at: www.toyl.
co.uk/pages/the-book

This list is about what makes you feel alive, what makes your life worth living. A Power Decade is a place of adventure, love, laughs, being uncomfortable as you try something new, being thrilled and celebrating when you achieve that something new, being open to success and failure. Travel, a new hobby, a new skill, going back to art school, doing an Open University course, starting a business, changing career, making new friends, finding new partners, moving home, straightening finances out, learning Latin dance in Argentina, learning to ride – what is it that would make you feel alive?

To make your life's dreams a reality, you have to plan them in, breaking them down into stages so that you achieve the big picture through baby steps every day.

This is how I do it:

Things you want to achieve? This is an open list because you can put anything and as many things as you want in here. You can add to it at any time, then plan new achievements.

Ten-Year Plan? This is the dream. In ten years' time, you want to be there or thereabouts. Again, put anything you want here.

Five-Year Plan – create this after the ten years as this should be about half way to your ten year goal. What does half way look like?

One-Year Plan – so, breaking the five-year plan down further, what can you achieve in the next year towards that final goal?

That was easy, wasn't it? But now you have to make it happen.

Before we go any further, check that you have all of these things in your Power Decade plan:

Something creative just for you. Art, drama, history, knitting, anything, but you have to have real, genuine creative time for you, not just half an hour in front of the TV. Adding in a creative element will be so good for you. Personally, I'm writing a book about a series of road trips that I'm taking around the UK on odd weekends when I have time. This means I have to visit places and research them before I go. I then have to write it up – fantastic! I couldn't be happier. It's highly likely no one will ever read that book, but I love it.

This is so important as being creative stimulates different brain cells to those we use otherwise, it makes us a more rounded person. You also have to differen-tiate being creative from having a hobby. Knitting is creative AND a hobby, rambling – lovely though it is – is just a hobby, there's a difference. You may not think you are any good at anything creative, it may not be something you naturally want to do but trust me, it is key to living well, however magnificent or not the results are, it's all to do with using different parts of your brain.

Did you put in exercise, nutrition and personal health? Go on, no need to create a plan as, frankly, I've told you what you need to do but there's a fitness plan at the back of the book and on my website if you want to use it.

Does any of it go beyond your current budget? OK, we need to find the cash for it, but that bit will also be fun.

Volunteering – don't miss this out, four hours per month.

Career – if your dreams involve your career, we need to talk about this.

Your dreams

Take a look at your list. How's it looking? I want you to reread everything you included in it and ask yourself a few things:

Do you really want it? Do you want to spend time achieving it? Some things are non-negotiable such as exercise, nutrition, being creative and volunteering, but the things you wrote down, the things that came from your core, are they still real for you? You're going to be spending a decade of time and effort striving for these things, so are you really sure? Take a few days to ponder them.

Be hard on yourself, are your goals genuinely realistic? By this, I'm not asking you to limit yourself, but if you've written 'Be the next Mrs Brad Pitt', you could be on a hiding to nothing. Just check that your dreams are all a stretch for you, but entirely possible given the right circumstances.

Think about you in ten years' time. If you have achieved what you've written down, will you think back on your life as fulfilled, well-lived? If not, revisit the goals. We are doing this so you can go into old age satisfied, looking back on a life well-lived, where you gave it your all.

Is your list balanced? When I first did mine, it was all about career, which isn't healthy. The compulsory additions of exercise, nutrition, volunteer work and a creative hobby are there to help the balance stay strong, but you *must* add in something for yourself, something you've always wanted to do. This could be education, travel, anything, but you cannot just have work (or finance) related goals; these will not make you happy in isolation.

Once you've examined the list, edited it, added to it and deleted from it until you are happy with it, it's time to divide the ambitions up.

Money. In this, list all the dreams you will need additional funds to make happen. Dreams can cross over into several boxes, but start by moving them into the category you think is most relevant.

Time. Does your dream need you to dedicate additional time to make it happen? If so, pop it in this box.

New skills. Does your dream require new skills? For example, if you want to change career, you may need different qualifications. If you want to live in Italy, you may need to learn the language. This is the place for those dreams.

Have a look at your dreams and ponder which ones seem to be the most difficult right now. Ask yourself why they seem to be the most difficult. Is it because funds are tight, is it because you have no time, or is it because you don't have the skills? Whichever dreams seem to be the most difficult will take the longest to achieve, so we can start them right now.

Using what you've just done, list your dreams in order of which ones you think will be the most difficult to achieve (still no 'Mrs Brad Pitt', please). Number one will be the most challenging, the lower ones less challenging. Take a moment to have a look at the list – is it right? Are you seeing difficulties where there aren't any? What we are going to do is make all those challenges, every one of them, go away. They are not real. You may think they are, but every one of them is solvable. It just depends on you taking action.

Putting to one side for now all the compulsory stuff (volunteering, nutrition, exercise, creative outlet), let's focus on what *you* wrote rather than me for a change. How do you feel now you've written your dreams down? Empowered and excited or daunted and depressed? If it's the latter, look at why you feel this way. It's all to do with your self-confidence, so the start of your personal Power Decade is going to be characterised by getting your self-confidence up because you need to be feeling empowered and excited by seeing the start of your dreams coming true, not down in the mouth. Write down self-confidence in year one and then break it down into what you are going to do each month and week to work on this, for example read books, work on positive affirmation, get professional help.

Excellent, now we can get cracking. Assuming that you are excited, let's make those challenges go away.

Money

Let's do two things. First, let's quantify how much money each of your dreams would be likely to need if you were to do them today. Second, let's take a long, hard look at your financial position. If money is an issue in making your dreams come true, it's likely that you don't have enough of it. Assuming that is so, let's start with the stuff that might be worrying you.

Debt

Have you got debt? Well, we need to make this go away because we don't want you getting into old age with debt, plus you will need money to make your dreams happen and you can't spend money on dreams if you have debt. I sound like my mother.

Midlife is a time for a few hard decisions. We need to get into financial shape. The Power Decade needs it, old age demands it, so we have to look this one in the face and call it an adventure, however it makes us feel.

If you have financial challenges, there are two places I'd go. First, I'd get an independent financial advisor (IFA) in, a good one who has been recommended to you. For me, an IFA managed to get my mortgage payments down by 70% each month for the same type of mortgage. They did the same for a friend who was almost besides herself with worry about her mortgage. Personally, I was happy to pay their fee. IFAs also don't judge.

Second, if you have credit card debts, call Citizen's Advice for help. They are experts in negotiating with credit card companies on your behalf and will come up with deals that could halt interest in its tracks. View this as a three- to five-year part of your Power Decade, but it needs to be dealt with. After your debts are gone, you can start putting money towards your dreams.

You may not have debt, but you just don't have any spare cash for dreams. We can get to this later.

For me, I've had enough financial hoo-ha in my life to last me well into old age. It was stressful, horrible, blighted my life and made me feel sick most days. But the fear of it, what we say to ourselves in our heads, is way more damaging than the reality. We think of what could happen, and before we've even picked up the phone, in our minds we've made ourselves homeless and in debtor's jail. Not good.

You must tackle *all* financial concerns as a priority. Today. You're not the first and you won't be the last to get into trouble with money, but my gosh, will you feel better to have a reasonable financial plan in place.

If you have a mortgage, this may be playing on your mind. Bluntly, your options are to pay it off, accept that you're going to have a mortgage into old age (and that's fine), sell and downsize, or sell and move into rented accommodation. If you choose the fourth option, you may have to work into old age to pay your rent, but you might have to do that anyway if you keep going with your mortgage. Decide what you want to do.

Personally, I'm all for attempting to pay a mortgage off, but the world's not a perfect place and we all have to accept that this may not happen, so let's look at both increasing our income later and making savings now to push mortgage payments downwards and give us more cash to take out in the long run. Many people go for an equity release plan in old age where they get to stay in their home, but it will then be partly owned by a company in return for them getting a lump sum, mortgage or not.

Are you willing to sacrifice or delay parts of your Power Decade plan to ensure that you have a bit more financial security? Be careful. In midlife, if you make the cut-back regime too rigid, there is far less potential for your dreams to happen on a regular basis, and you're time limited now. Being really blunt, you don't want to find that life has dealt you an unexpected blow health wise and all you've got to show is a bit more financial security rather than a life well-lived. But if you can cut back a bit, do. It'll be worth it. Sensible financial planning – there are enough apps out there to help you with monthly household expense planning and enough people to help you with debt – will put you in a better mental space. Details are listed at the end of the book but remember, I'm not a financial advisor so if you need professional help, get it.

Now we've got through the lack of finances, how are we going to increase our income? Two ways – promotion to a better job or take a second job, which may be our own business.

Promotion

Think you're 'too old' for promotion? Stop it.

Oh my goodness, this is one of the most fantastic things. In midlife, your career is completely open to you. You can do anything you want, so if you do want a career change, now is your moment. Isn't this just incredibly exciting?

I changed career at the age of fifty-two and it is the best thing I have ever done. I'm now engaged with the job, motivated, excited, meeting amazing people, doing things that scare me a lot, doing things that humble me with the bravery, kindness and compassion of the people I meet. I'm not sure what else I'd want from a working life, but it wasn't always that way.

I was in beauty PR for twenty-five years. The journalists were fine and I love the beauty industry (which is what I specialised in), but I found it fairly soul destroying. Running Time of Your Life, my beauty subscription box, is an absolute passion. I love the podcasts, the blogs, the speaking, curating the box, the suppliers I talk to, the writing, the videos – I love it all, even the days when it all goes to hell in a handcart.

That's how you should feel. So, how are we going to get you there?

If you're in a company and you want promotion, you are going to have to work for it. If promotion isn't possible, you're going to have to look at moving to a company offering better pay. If you're in a company and have no chance of promotion because of lack of qualifications, you're going to have to get qualified.

All of these are challenging, but completely doable if that's what you want.

Getting promotion means looking the part for the job you want before you get it. It's the 'fake it till you make it' concept. I'd advise letting your boss know that you want promotion and an increased salary (you don't just want the job title, that's not what this is about), and ask their advice on how to get it. This puts it in their mind to consider you from that day onwards as someone who wants to move up in the world.

Secondly, you're going to have to take on extra jobs and responsibility now. Show your boss that you're serious. Send a message that you can do the job, but be aware that this can be a risky strategy. Your boss might be mean enough to say, 'Ho well, if you're going to take on an increased workload without the position or pay rise, happy days.' Limit this period to a maximum of six months, after which you need to be brave enough to apply to other companies or confront your boss's boss about this.

You may also need new qualifications to get promotion and a pay rise. If so, find out which the best qualifications are and make a start. It's an extra drain on your time, but there's a reason people get paid more for certain roles, and it's because they studied for extra skills. Accept this, knuckle down and crack on. You are likely to find studying again immensely rewarding – I know I did, and I was very sniffy about what any course might be able to teach me. I was wrong and I'm on one course or another most of the time these days. It opens my mind.

Second job

Here's where I'd like you to think about boxing a bit more cleverly. If you need more cash, you can take a second job. This limits your time, but it can be incredibly rewarding. You can also consider setting up a business, perhaps with a friend, and for this I'd suggest an internet business because start-up is so cheap.

I was on one of the many social-media platforms yesterday – this one dedicated to business – and a comment came up from a well-known 'business angel' who deserves to be named and shamed, but I've done legal before and it's not within my current bank balance to do so again. Anyway, the point he was making was that he would never invest money in a business run by anyone (man or woman) over forty as they just don't have the energy.

Where do I start on this one? In midlife, aren't we the ones running everything, from our jobs to our kids to our parents to our partners, from running the home to getting in the exercise, from planning holidays to sorting out the bills, from purchasing stuff to keeping the home together? Exactly what bit of 'no energy' applies to us? But the problem you and I have is that, frankly, this 'business angel' doesn't value this type of work because it cannot be quantified in monetary terms. All midlife women cope with amazing workloads and our efforts are quietly unacknowledged by everyone but our families (and our families only if we're lucky). That's the prejudice we face.

If you have yearned to run your own business, now is the time to do it. If we look at the *Harvard Business Review* stats and not the comments of a middle-aged man, a start-up business has way more success if it's launched by a fifty-year-old than a twenty-something year old. In fact, the average age of a successful start-up entrepreneur is forty-five, so why don't you do it? Do it now, while the odds are in your favour, and yes, you *do* still have the energy to run it well. It doesn't matter if your ambitions are big or small, full-time or part-time, it will be an amazing experience and one – if you manage it well – you are unlikely to regret.

The fantastic thing about the era we live in is that anyone can run a great business from their sofa in their pants (not that I do, you understand). The internet and social media make access to market incredibly simple, but it isn't simple to get it right. I'm personally not a great one for business plans (unless you're trying to get investment) because in my long experience, most business plans are like war plans – shot to hell in the first contact with the market, and then you're making it up as you go along and using your instinct to try to get it right. All entrepreneurs have great failure stories to tell, but all of this failure led them to be more successful the day after because they learned from it.

You are a bright, intelligent woman who understands risk, what feels right and what feels wrong. That's pretty much all you need to start a business. If you want any further advice, don't hesitate to email me on info@toyl.co.uk and you can have all the benefit of my knowledge, but if your own business is your ambition, go for it!

While we're at it, I would also refer you to the health section. If you're going to run your own business, you will need all the energy you can get as the hours are long and the work taxing, both mentally and physically, at least at the start. Get yourself in shape. I know, but it's a drum I'm going to keep on banging.

If you want to start an internet shop (because if you want a second income, you're likely to have to sell stuff), then I recommend Shopify as it is a ready-made online shop and has a free Shopify academy that you can access without being a Shopify customer. Here, the world's best internet sellers give free online videos and courses on marketing, working your site, making it easy for visitors to get around your site – all of it. I've used other platforms as well, but I've found Shopify to be the best.

If you don't want to run an online business, think about alternatives. It could be direct selling a product such as Avon, where the business model is already in place for you. There are so many options for these type of businesses, from jewellery to cosmetics, kitchenware to wine, meal plans to food supplements. Don't believe all the negatives you hear about these businesses, there are some quality companies out there and the start-up is simple. Do a bit of research and perhaps begin with a party for your friends. I'm sure they would love to support you. Don't dismiss having your own online business on the side of your regular job, but before you start, upgrade your computer and phone to work with the latest versions of social media and computer software or you'll struggle.

I hope this section has opened your eyes to the fact that there are options for solving debt, reducing your outgoings and increasing your income. It's in no way definitive, but research will lead you to your answers. Open your mind.

Savings

Once you've got the debt under control and found some spare cash from promotion, a second job or cuts in budgets, you need to start saving to make your dreams happen. Only you know how expensive your dreams will be, but I suggest getting an app designed for savings, putting money into an account (or accounts) and using the app to plan how much money to allocate for each dream. If you're saving £50 a month, it could be £10 for your trip to see the gorillas in Borneo, £20 towards a course you really want to do and £20 towards a dating agency so you can meet the partner of your dreams. You get the idea, and see the list of apps at the end of the book.

What if you look at what you can save and it's not enough, by any stretch, to make your dreams happen? If you've done all you can to help yourself, but there's just no further slack in the system. With this, you need to be realistic. Look at your dreams. Is there a slightly less expensive version of any of them that you could accept? Some maybe, some maybe not, but have a look.

It's worth asking your IFA about where to put your savings. If your dream is a trip with the grandchildren to Florida and it is several years away, your IFA may know of a scheme that pays better dividends than keeping your money in the bank. Ask advice. You don't have to take it.

You cannot dip into your savings, so you need to have an everyday fund as well for clothes, weekends away etc. Make sure your monthly budget has a separate savings account so that your dream fund is sacrosanct. The rule of thumb is to spend no more than 5% of your net pay on clothes, which may seem rather mean for most of us, but we've probably all got too many clothes anyway.

Finances are tricky to look at because all of our circumstances are different, but we need to take control of them for our own sake, regardless of who does what in our household.

Time

'I just want one day off when I can go swimming and eat ice cream and look at rainbows.'
—Mariah Carey, singer and superstar

This is a quote from a woman who works very hard. I know I've cut into your available time, but I'm making you engage in the world a lot more. You're now exercising, eating well, spending time being creative and volunteering. You might also be studying, running a second business or working longer hours to get promotion. But how do you get the time to fulfil your dreams?

Here's the good news. The likelihood is that everything I've asked you to do, you will be enjoying. These activities may even have become part of your dreams. Being healthy is a fantastic thing, giving your time is amazing, and being creative feeds your soul. Dreams are the icing on the cake, and most dreams start in year one with the basics I've outlined, so you get to live a great life straight away. And if you've found time to get those basics into your life, you can find the time to make your dreams come true.

One of my dreams is to be living in sunny climates during the winter. I get ill every winter in the UK and it's not good, so sun would be great. This requires four months away, but actually, most of the basics I can do abroad – exercise, eat well, volunteer, be creative. Sure, I need finances to support three to four months elsewhere while covering costs at home, but there are many places in the world where it's hot in winter and incredibly cheap to live. I just need to make it happen.

You're a motivated person if you are putting your Power Decade plan into action, so find a way. Oprah, Michelle Obama and Beyoncé all have the same twenty-four hours as you. Yes, they have help, but they didn't always; they just powered through. In midlife we have as much energy as we had in our twenties, fact. Find the time if it's important to you.

New skills

When I reached fifty, I thought I knew it all. Frankly, I thought I knew it all at eighteen, but at fifty, I *really* thought I knew it all. But of course, I didn't.

One of the biggest mistakes you can make in midlife is to stop learning. If you need to study for work, do it. Even Kim Kardashian is apparently studying to become a lawyer, with all her millions in the bank. She wants to be able to help people who've experienced miscarriages of justice (see, another one volunteering with actions, not cash. Cash is not what the world needs from us). I have no doubt she feels empowered by what she is learning. Exhausted, but empowered.

Your Power Decade needs to be packed with learning new skills to achieve your dreams, so don't shy away from it. If you take up an Open University course, you will meet some amazing students who will help you through. If you're mending fences on the Cornish costal path, you're likely to be thrilled at who you meet and the beauty of nature. Learning new skills taught me so much about myself that it was worth it just for that.

Embrace learning – the fear, the subject matter, the self-consciousness, all of it. Embrace it and take everything it can give you.

The plan

We've tackled the key issues of achieving our Power Decade, now we need to pull all our bits of paper together. Start with this:

Where do I see myself in five years' time? This is a smaller version of the ten-year plan. Put in where you think you can be in your journey towards your goals here.

Where do I see myself in one year's time? This is where you have to see a tenth of your dream come true. Here, plan the goals that will be achievable in one year's time that will work towards your ten-year goal. You already know some of the challenges or advantages the next year will hold, so the planning should already be pretty good. Make your one-year plan achievable.

What do I need to do to get there? Here's where you list whatever skills you might need to achieve your goals, anyone you need to find to help you, like a great IFA, a voluntary organisation you love or a group to encourage you lose weight or work on your happiness. Make a note of how you might find these people.

How does that look on a monthly basis? Break your one-year programme down into what you are going to achieve each month.

How does that look on a weekly basis? This could just be time you need to block out for work on your dreams, or it could be getting rid of stuff. Look at it all. Build this time into your weekly schedule, the same as food shopping, the same as work, the same as time with your friends. You won't achieve the ten-year plan without this weekly work.

Now all you have to do is do it.

What can you expect from your power decade?

'You don't come into this life wanting to be anything other than happy.'
—Demi Moore, fifty-six, actress

Peace of mind. Knowledge that life has not passed you by. Fulfilment of your dreams. Happiness. That's what you are doing this for.

Before your forties, the things that made you happy were likely to have been travel, adventure, shopping, romance – the usual standbys that Instagram sells to us. In midlife, your Power Decade is about trying to achieve what you think will make you happy while you still have the time and energy. Let's see if we can find happiness by stretching, reaching and growing. In short, it's time to choose to be happy through deeds, thoughts and actions.

Goodness knows, Demi Moore has had her share of challenges, what with Ashton and all, yet I'm in awe of the Zen-like way that she chooses to live her life, fighting the negative thoughts that, surely, she must have about some of the situations she's been in. Bitterness can eat you up and destroy any chance of happiness, but only if you let it. Demi chooses happiness, and I want that for you.

Here I've listed five things that a thirty-year-old may typically believe will make them happy:

1. A million quid

2. Diamonds

3. Mortgage paid off

4. Better body

5. Better husband/partner's body

Any of these look familiar? OK, look closely at the list and ask yourself whether they would really make you happy in midlife. Redo the list and see if it doesn't look a bit more like this:

1. Kids sorted, in jobs, not doing drugs, going along OK

2. Family health good

3. Time to do a project you've always wanted to do

4. Happy partner relationship

5. Money sorted

The thing is, you've had at least twenty years of working to get the bling in the first list, and if you did it, great. If, like most of us, you messed around, thinking time was eternal, then you've got to accept that you now have to prioritise, and diamonds just aren't part of that list. Trust me, I bought and sold the same diamond ten years apart for exactly the same price – it hadn't gone up in value at all, whereas a happy partner relationship/ good health/happy family pays you back tenfold. The key is not just to do something for yourself, although that's important, but to ensure that your loved ones and community are going along OK too. There is incredible happiness in that.

So that's it, then. Your midlife years can be the most amazing, fulfilling, meteoric time of your life. Sure, there's a bit of work to do on your health, but once you have that nailed, the world is literally yours *if you put your plan into action.*

Always remember:

- You, a midlife woman, are part of the fastest growing demographic worldwide

- You control 67% of all consumer spend in your household (possibly more)

- You control 80% of healthcare decisions for your loved ones

- You could put a whole week's worth of your amazing skills into your favourite projects for global good every year if you volunteered for just four hours per month

Together, we can literally change the world. Use your power for good.

You and I are preparing to say goodbye for now. You have your plan for your Power Decade and, perhaps unknown to you, you also have the wisdom to put it into action. You have unbelievable life skills and you have the ability to put these to work for your own good, your family's good and the good of your community. Do so. No regrets. Live well. Don't wait. As Oprah says, 'If not now, when?' The time is now. Crack on, meet your Power Decade head on.

We, those a bit further down the road, are all here; we're on the parade route with our flags waving, shouting your success on. There's a party later with all of us, but this part of the parade is just for you; it's all about you, so don't miss it. Own it; show us how you are going to set light to this time in your life. Stride out in your parade, help others along the way, show us what a strong, compassionate, generous and engaged-with-the-world woman you are. Pick your best party outfit, meet new friends, link hands and take the first step on the journey. Can you hear the crowd roar to welcome you? Can you feel their support? Of course you can because it's all of us in the crowd, lifting you up, guiding you, willing you on. We're all waiting at the end of parade party to celebrate you.

I'll see you there.

Further Resources

I have *no* sponsorship at all from any of the companies I recommend below. I purchase all their goods or services at full price, just like any other regular customer, and none of them knew they'd end up in this book until I asked their permission.

You don't have to go with my choices at all, I'm sure you're bright enough to find your own favourites, but these are things that I like. For ease, all the web links are also on my website at www.toyl.co.uk/book_resources

The Time of Your Life doesn't end here.

Weight Watchers and Slimming World

You might not need them, but I've been members of both and they do help. First, you get to record your food and the quantities you eat, which is key to knowing where you are overeating. Then the shame of the weigh-in focuses your mind like nothing else. There's also the sanctimonious euphoria when you do lose weight. Finally, most people at these groups are kindness personified. I use the Weight Watchers' app, it really helps me to see how greedy I'm being and rein back my portion size. Of course, there are other groups to help you lose weight, so try them out to find what works for you.

www.weightwatchers.com

www.slimmingworld.co.uk

Omega fatty acid test kit

Dr Glenville, mentioned in the book, has spent a life-time caring about and looking at women's health through nutrition, so she gets my money every time. You can find out how to obtain your test kit at www. naturalhealthpractice.com/Omega_3_Finger_Prick_ Deficie_P1980C348.cfm

Vitamin supplements

Gosh, aren't there loads on the market? I've used these in the past, mainly because I think they care about the manufacturing, but really choose to suit your body and pocket:

www.holfordirect.com

These are created by Dr Patrick Holford who has a really strong pedigree in creating great vitamin supplements.

www.naturalhealthpractice.com

Dr Glenville has spent her whole life looking at women's health through diet and supplements so I trust her to deliver great products.

Pelvic floor exercises

The UK National Health Service has a fantastic app called Squeezy. At the time of writing it is £2.99 and works on most smartphones.

I've actually purchased an Elvie (available from www. elvie.com and John Lewis in the UK) which is also app-run and a bit more expensive at £169 (at the time of writing).

It doesn't really matter which you go for, but do pelvic floor exercises – you'll thank me later in life (again…).

Bone density scan

If you're under seventy-five you can't just ask for a bone density scan in the UK on the NHS, you have to be at risk. If your mum or sister has been diagnosed then go from your early fifties and ask for a scan, they can but say no. If you want one privately they cost around £75 currently.

If you have a heel bone density scan this isn't going to be as accurate as a hip and back scan, called a DXA or DEXA scan, but it is going to be a lot cheaper and it will give you an idea. If this comes up with a worrying result go to your doctor to get the full DXA scan.

Osteoporosis is a real challenge for women and just because you are unaffected now please don't assume you won't be. Visit the National Osteoporosis Society to find out more: www.nos.org.uk

Menopause books

Where do we start? Menopause books are a recent phenomenon and, as I write, some woman somewhere is writing what will become our definitive guide. In the meantime my favourite practical book is:

Making Friends with the Menopause by Sarah Rayner and Dr Patrick Fitzgerald (2015, CreateSpace Independent Publishing Platform)

This next book is really good to understand the transition from perimenopause into full menopause:

The Perimenopause Handbook by Andrea Glover (2018, Xlibris, UK)

Then this book helps you to understand how your diet impacts you to get through the menopause well:

Natural Solutions to Menopause by Dr Marilyn Glenville (2011, Bluebird, London)

Finally, if you want some 'girl power' and sympathy from others that have been this way you can either go with Andrea McLean or Germaine Greer, depending on your preference:

Confessions of a Menopausal Woman by Andrea McLean (2019, Corgi Press, London)

The Change by Germaine Greer (2019, Bloomsbury Publishing, London)

I also have to give a shout out to www.megsmenopause. com. Run by Meg Matthews, she is one of the first on Instagram and her website to shout out about the menopause, and she also hosts an annual conference with a bevy of fantastic speakers who can help. Follow her.

Menopausal mental health help

Take this seriously and if you have any mental health issues that you cannot resolve quickly please go and see your GP as soon as you can. Your mental health is key to your wellness and if you think you have any concerns around this at all, take a look at these sites:

www.nhs.uk/conditions/menopause

This is the NHS site in the UK where you can find out about the link between the menopause and mental health.

www.healthline.com/health/menopause/mental-health

This site talks about how to recognise the symptoms and some simple changes you can make to help.

www.mentalhealth.org.uk/tags/menopause

This is a mental health organisation's take on what you can do to help yourself.

Menopause home test

These are all over the internet and range in price from about £10 to £30. I'd suggest the one from Superdrug (www.superdrug.com) because it's a name we know and trust. All of them are blood tests so follow the instructions well to get a clear result and answer the questions honestly. If you are perimenopausal then it's worth getting checked over by your doctor just to discuss how you feel and any issues that have come up. Remember, I struggled with period flooding for years because I assumed that I just had to suffer this rather than going to see the doctor to get it sorted. Don't be as dumb as me, it's your health so look after yourself.

Changing your mindset

If that little voice in your head isn't talking nicely to you, here are some books that might help it change its attitude pronto.

The Mind Makeover by Sharron Lowe (2014, Piatkus, London)

Change Your Life in 7 Days by Paul McKenna (2004, Bantum Press, London)

The Chimp Paradox by Steve Peters (2012, Vermilion, London)

Volunteer organisations

These are myriad so go looking for them. There is something for everyone, from organic farming to beach clear ups, NHS volunteering to helping kids. Here are some ideas to get you started:

www.gov.uk/government/get-involved/take-part/volunteer

www.ncvo.org.uk/ncvo-volunteering/i-want-to-volunteer

www.ivsgb.org/guide-to-volunteering-in-the-uk

UK volunteering holidays

I haven't been on any of these, but I fancy them! All of these links enable you to get away for a few days, a week or longer:

www.nationaltrust.org.uk/holidays/working-holidays/search

wwoof.org.uk (organic farming opportunities)

www.waterways.org.uk/wrg/regional_groups/regional_groups

International volunteering holidays

I haven't been on any of these either, they cost more, but if it's your cup of tea to volunteer abroad check out these:

www.gvi.co.uk

www.andamandiscoveries.com

www.blacksheepinn.com

Financial planning apps

Disclaimer. I'm not a financial advisor and if you need real help please see a professional. In my opinion, these are good apps to help personal financial planning:

YOLT: helps you sync cards, bank accounts and savings accounts all together

Goodbudget Budget Planner: a money and expenses tracker

Money Monitor: expenses tracker

All of the above are on my website so you just need to click on the links or visit www.toyl.co.uk/pages/ the-book

Time Of Your Life Worksheets

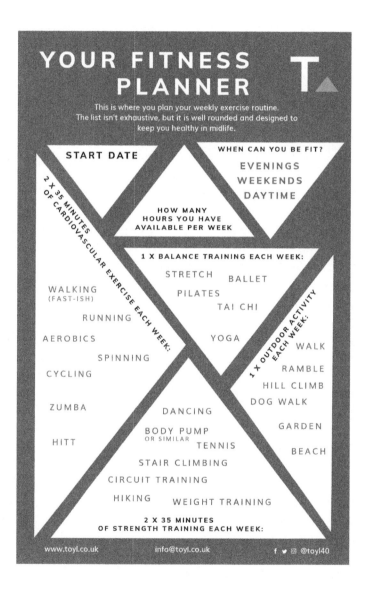

YOUR FITNESS PLANNER T▲

This is where you plan your weekly exercise routine.
The list isn't exhaustive, but it is well rounded and designed to keep you healthy in midlife.

START DATE

WHEN CAN YOU BE FIT?

EVENINGS
WEEKENDS
DAYTIME

HOW MANY HOURS YOU HAVE AVAILABLE PER WEEK

2 X 35 MINUTES OF CARDIOVASCULAR EXERCISE EACH WEEK:

1 X BALANCE TRAINING EACH WEEK:

STRETCH   BALLET

PILATES

TAI CHI

WALKING
(FAST-ISH)

RUNNING

YOGA

1 X OUTDOOR ACTIVITY EACH WEEK:

AEROBICS

SPINNING

WALK

CYCLING

RAMBLE

HILL CLIMB

DOG WALK

ZUMBA

DANCING

GARDEN

BODY PUMP
OR SIMILAR

TENNIS

HITT

BEACH

STAIR CLIMBING

CIRCUIT TRAINING

HIKING   WEIGHT TRAINING

2 X 35 MINUTES OF STRENGTH TRAINING EACH WEEK:

www.toyl.co.uk   info@toyl.co.uk   f 🐦 📷 @toyl40

T▲ MONTHLY QUIT CHART

I AM QUITTING _____

WHY? _____

Fill in the date and tick if you succeeded in quitting or put a cross if you didn't.

At th end ofthe month add up the no of ticks and put the total in bottom right box.

REPEAT EVERY MONTH.

START DATE

DATE   DATE

TOTAL NUMBER OF TICKS

REWARD

www.toyl.co.uk   info@toyl.co.uk   f ✈ ⓐ @toyl40

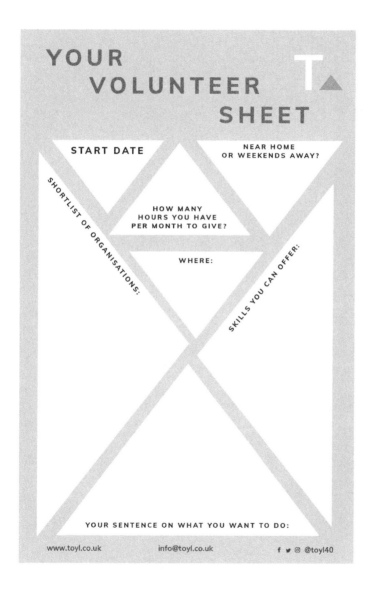

YOUR
VOLUNTEER
SHEET
T▲

START DATE

NEAR HOME
OR WEEKENDS AWAY?

SHORTLIST OF ORGANISATIONS:

HOW MANY
HOURS YOU HAVE
PER MONTH TO GIVE?

WHERE:

SKILLS YOU CAN OFFER:

YOUR SENTENCE ON WHAT YOU WANT TO DO:

www.toyl.co.uk   info@toyl.co.uk   f ♥ ◎ @toyl40

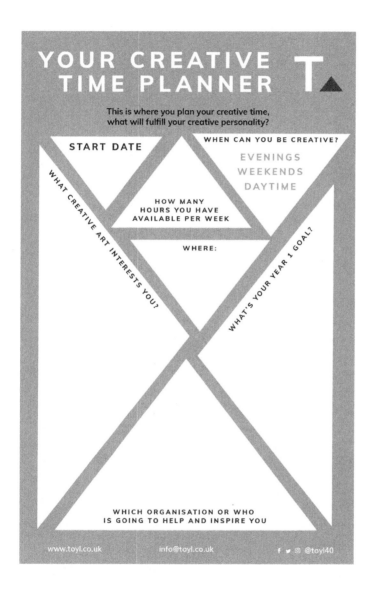

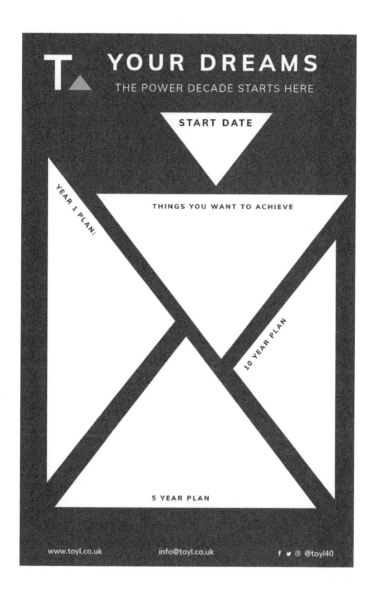

Acknowledgments

How long have you got? It took a lifetime to write this book so there are a few people right there.

Friends: I'd like to thank the Twiglets, Perks, Lav, JoJo and Carol. You put up with someone who is not easy.

Family: I'd like to thank all my in-laws for being kind as I know I'm tricky. My brothers and nephews just have to put up with me, but I love them for that.

My fellow volunteers: Ed, Hannah, John, Father Peter, Jenny and JoJo (again) for the fantastic work you do in our tiny little village and for putting up with my good (and sometimes hopeless) ideas with a kindness that never ceases to amaze me.

My business partner, Stuart, and John for listening. He keeps asking for a man's version of this book but that's one for him to write.

There are also women in the beauty industry who have been incredibly generous to me with their time. Lee Pycroft is an inspiration on Instagram every day; Sue Peart has taught me how to be open minded to new people, as she is; Tracey Woodward remains one of the most generous women in the industry; and Jo Morton, as I'm thankful every day for her longstanding friendship. Thank you all.

Finally, those at home. We're not big on sentiment in our family, we just all know, deep down, how tightly knit we are, how much we love each other and that we would be lost without each other. How lucky am I?

The Author

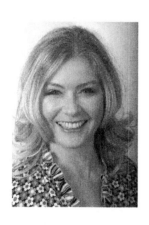Karen is an award-winning 40+ beauty blogger and an ex-beauty PR with over twenty years' experience, having created major beauty promotions for most of the UK media. She is the founder of Time of Your Life, a monthly subscription beauty box for midlife women which also offers podcasts and blogs on a range of subjects specifically targeted to women. Karen personally curates every box, choosing products specifically designed for women over forty.

She has as dysfunctional a family as any, has been divorced, had children, had businesses succeed and fail, had quite a few mammograms and has lost both parents. But, she's a firm believer that midlife women are the greatest force for good in the world, they just don't know their own power – yet.

Karen speaks around the UK and USA every year as she updates what she learns about midlife and how the world responds to midlife women, the fastest growing demographic on the planet. You can find out about her upcoming speaking dates and much more on the TOYL website or the company's social media.

On the website, you can also sign up to Karen's free weekly newsletter, blog and podcasts, which talk about issues for midlife women, stuff she's been up to, musings, beauty news and interviews with interesting people.

Connect with Karen, get involved and access the TOYL YouTube channel at: www.TOYL.co.uk

@toyl40

Time Of Your Life

@toyl40